The Role of Nutrition in ADHD, Psychiatric, and Mental Disorders Treatment

The Role of Nutrition in ADHD, Psychiatric, and Mental Disorders Treatment

Editors

Roser Granero
Diego Redolar-Ripoll

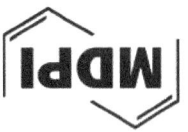

MDPI • Basel • Beijing • Wuhan • Barcelona • Belgrade • Manchester • Tokyo • Cluj • Tianjin

Editors
Roser Granero
Autonomous University
of Barcelona
Spain

Diego Redolar-Ripoll
UOC Universitat Oberta
de Catalunya
Spain

Editorial Office
MDPI
St. Alban-Anlage 66
4052 Basel, Switzerland

This is a reprint of articles from the Special Issue published online in the open access journal *Nutrients* (ISSN 2072-6643) (available at: https://www.mdpi.com/journal/nutrients/special_issues/Nutrition_ADHD).

For citation purposes, cite each article independently as indicated on the article page online and as indicated below:

LastName, A.A.; LastName, B.B.; LastName, C.C. Article Title. *Journal Name* **Year**, *Volume Number*, Page Range.

ISBN 978-3-0365-3397-1 (HbK)
ISBN 978-3-0365-3398-8 (PDF)

© 2022 by the authors. Articles in this book are Open Access and distributed under the Creative Commons Attribution (CC BY) license, which allows users to download, copy and build upon published articles, as long as the author and publisher are properly credited, which ensures maximum dissemination and a wider impact of our publications.

The book as a whole is distributed by MDPI under the terms and conditions of the Creative Commons license CC BY-NC-ND.

Contents

About the Editors vii

Roser Granero
Role of Nutrition and Diet on Healthy Mental State
Reprinted from: *Nutrients* **2022**, *14*, 750, doi:10.3390/nu14040750 1

Elisa Berthelot, Damien Etchecopar-Etchart, Dimitri Thellier, Christophe Lancon, Laurent Boyer and Guillaume Fond
Fasting Interventions for Stress, Anxiety and Depressive Symptoms: A Systematic Review and Meta-Analysis
Reprinted from: *Nutrients* **2021**, *13*, 3947, doi:10.3390/nu13113947 9

Julio Plaza-Diaz, Katherine Flores-Rojas, María José de la Torre-Aguilar, Antonio Rafael Gomez-Fernández, Pilar Martín-Borreguero, Juan Luis Perez-Navero, Angel Gil and Mercedes Gil-Campos
Dietary Patterns, Eating Behavior, and Nutrient Intakes of Spanish Preschool Children with Autism Spectrum Disorders
Reprinted from: *Nutrients* **2021**, *13*, 3551, doi:10.3390/nu13103551 23

Elena Yorgidis, Lisa Beiner, Nicola Blazynski, Katja Schneider-Momm, Hans-Willi Clement, Reinhold Rauh, Eberhard Schulz, Christina Clement and Christian Fleischhaker
Individual Behavioral Reactions in the Context of Food Sensitivities in Children with Attention-Deficit/Hyperactivity Disorder before and after an Oligoantigenic Diet
Reprinted from: *Nutrients* **2021**, *13*, 2598, doi:10.3390/nu13082598 41

Javier C. Vázquez, Ona Martin de la Torre, Júdit López Palomé and Diego Redolar-Ripoll
Effects of Caffeine Consumption on Attention Deficit Hyperactivity Disorder (ADHD) Treatment: A Systematic Review of Animal Studies
Reprinted from: *Nutrients* **2022**, *14*, 739, doi:10.3390/nu14040739 59

Monique Aucoin, Laura LaChance, Umadevi Naidoo, Daniella Remy, Tanisha Shekdar, Negin Sayar, Valentina Cardozo, Tara Rawana, Irina Chan and Kieran Cooley
Diet and Anxiety: A Scoping Review
Reprinted from: *Nutrients* **2021**, *13*, 4418, doi:10.3390/nu13124418 83

Roser Granero, Alfred Pardo-Garrido, Ivonne Lorena Carpio-Toro, Andrés Alexis Ramírez-Coronel, Pedro Carlos Martínez-Suárez and Geovanny Genaro Reivan-Ortiz
The Role of Iron and Zinc in the Treatment of ADHD among Children and Adolescents: A Systematic Review of Randomized Clinical Trials
Reprinted from: *Nutrients* **2021**, *13*, 4059, doi:10.3390/nu13114059 107

Mina Nicole Händel, Jeanett Friis Rohde, Marie Louise Rimestad, Elisabeth Bandak, Kirsten Birkefoss, Britta Tendal, Sanne Lemcke and Henriette Edemann Callesen
Efficacy and Safety of Polyunsaturated Fatty Acids Supplementation in the Treatment of Attention Deficit Hyperactivity Disorder (ADHD) in Children and Adolescents: A Systematic Review and Meta-Analysis of Clinical Trials
Reprinted from: *Nutrients* **2021**, *13*, 1226, doi:10.3390/nu13041226 127

About the Editors

Roser Granero has a PhD in Psychology (Autonomous University of Barcelona, AUB, since 1998), University Diploma in Statistics since 1997, Master in Design and Statistics in Behavioral Sciences since 2000, and Master in Child and Adolescent Psychopathology since 1997. Professor at the Psychobiology and Methodology Department of the AUB since 2001. Researcher at the CIBERobn Group (Center for Biomedical Research in Network for Obesity and Nutrition, Instituto Carlos III, Spain) and at the Department of Psychiatry of the University Hospital of Bellvitge (Barcelona, Spain). With more than 270 published research studies. Research area: design, statistics, and methodology for scientific analysis in health sciences, eating disorders and behavioral addictions.

Diego Redolar-Ripoll is an Associate Professor of Neuroscience and Psychobiology and Vice-Dean of Research in the Department of Psychology and Educational Sciences at the Universitat Oberta de Catalunya (UOC). His research focuses on the study of cognitive control using non-invasive brain stimulation techniques. Specifically, his interest focuses on the neural dissociation of two brain networks that integrate different portions of the prefrontal cortex, namely, a dorsal network that includes the dorsolateral part and a ventral network that includes the ventrolateral part.

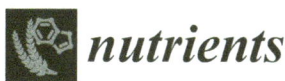

Editorial

Role of Nutrition and Diet on Healthy Mental State

Roser Granero [1,2,3]

[1] Department of Psychobiology and Methodology, Autonomous University of Barcelona, 08193 Barcelona, Spain; Roser.granero@uab.cat
[2] Ciber Fisiopatología Obesidad y Nutrición (CIBERobn), Instituto Salud Carlos III, 28015 Madrid, Spain
[3] Psychoneurobiology of Eating and Addictive Behaviors Group, Neurosciences Programme, Bellvitge Biomedical Research Institute (IDIBELL), 08908 Barcelona, Spain

Citation: Granero, R. Role of Nutrition and Diet on Healthy Mental State. *Nutrients* 2022, 14, 750. https://doi.org/10.3390/nu14040750

Received: 9 January 2022
Accepted: 7 February 2022
Published: 10 February 2022

Publisher's Note: MDPI stays neutral with regard to jurisdictional claims in published maps and institutional affiliations.

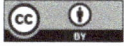

Copyright: © 2022 by the author. Licensee MDPI, Basel, Switzerland. This article is an open access article distributed under the terms and conditions of the Creative Commons Attribution (CC BY) license (https://creativecommons.org/licenses/by/4.0/).

1. Introduction

A large number of scientists and health professionals recognize that balanced nutrition is fundamental for a good state of physical health. The World Health Organization working group focused on nutrition as a key component of disease prevention, indicating that *"a balanced and varied diet, composed of a wide range of nutritious and tasty foods, adds years to life and life to years"* [1]. In their report, this group also warns that a high percentage of common diseases in industrialized countries (such as obesity, diabetes, hypertension, coronary heart disease and even certain cancers) are directly or indirectly related to inefficient nutrition, especially with the elevated intake of processed foods high in trans-fatty acids and low consumption of essential nutrients (mainly vitamins, minerals and proteins). The 13th General Programme of Work approved by the Health Assembly during May 2018 (GPW13) [2], was developed to guide the work team of WHO during 2019–2023, providing priority actions to promote wellbeing during the lifetime (the key element being the reduction of salt/sodium intake and industrialy produced trans-fat) and encouraging the support of the Member States with a roadmap for countries [3].

However, a greater controversy exists in the scientific community regarding the role of nutrition on the onset and progression of mental diseases and behavioral problems, and it is unclear how diet may contribute to therapeutic efficiency regarding patients with diverse psychopathological states. Unfortunately, strategies based on making diet changes and sticking with them are often overlooked in treatments for mental health conditions.

In the following sections, we review current studies that analyze the role of specific diet components in the interventions addressed for common mental disorders in developed countries among children and adolescents. Since the psychopathologies considered in this review have elevated risk of comorbid health hazards, the evidence-based interventions for psychiatric patients covering proper nutrition could promote large-scale physical and mental wellbeing. Furthermore, the results of these intervention programs could provide the basis for developing targeted disease prevention programs aimed to reduce modifiable risk factors.

2. Diet Intervention on ADHD

Attention-deficit/hyperactivity disorder (ADHD) is a chronic neurodevelopmental disorder whose etiology is the result of complex interactions between multiple factors, including genetic, biological and environmental influences. The disorder is usually diagnosed when a child is of school age, with a worldwide prevalence estimate of 6% during childhood [4], and persistent into adulthood with a mean rate of 43% (estimates between adults is around 3% within population-based samples) [5]. Several harmful consequences are associated with ADHD, including deficient academic/work performance, social isolation, aggressive behavior (including delinquency and illegal acts) and even premature death from unnatural causes (such as accidents) [6].

The standard intervention for ADHD combines pharmacological treatment (largely psychostimulants) with psychological therapy. The beneficial short-term efficacy of such treatments in reducing acute core symptoms is largely verified, but the long-term effects are not clearly evidenced: most patients may still show ADHD symptoms and may not attain normalized behavior even with combined medication and behavioral therapy, which results in frequent medication nonadherence (around 50% within months 12 to 36 of the follow-up). Current studies on alternative interventions for ADHD aim at the prevention of ADHD progression and targeting the underlying triggers (such as stress, poor sleep, overstimulation, technology or dietary plans). On the basis that making adequate lifestyle changes to minimize these triggers could contribute to better control of ADHD symptoms, studies addressing the efficacy of nutrition on the developmental course of ADHD have observed that deficiencies in certain types of foods can worsen the symptoms of attention deficit, hyperactivity and impulsivity, while adequate dietary plans could optimize brain functions. Most of these treatment studies are focused on exploring the role of vitamins, minerals and polyunsaturated fatty acids [7], with controversial results depending on diverse factors (i.e., sample composition, measurement tools or diet components).

Results obtained by a current systematic review reinforce the effectiveness of ADHD treatments with complementary diet interventions, although the benefits could be different for subgroups of patients with different profiles. Concretely, the study of Granero and colleagues [8] focused on the contribution of iron and zinc supplementation in the progression of ADHD among children and adolescents, observed in randomized trials published during the last two decades. The conclusion was that at baseline (before the treatment), low zinc and iron levels were associated with higher symptom levels (particularly with attention capacity and hyperactivity behavior), suggesting a pathway mediated by the dopaminergic system. Additionally, regarding the contribution to the treatment of ADHD, it was observed that zinc supplementation consistently improved and compensated baseline borderline zinc nutrition, contributing to improvements in most ADHD cases. However, the role of iron supplementation was more inconsistent, and it seemed that its benefits are centered specifically in children with low ferritin/iron stores at baseline, as restoring adequate levels contributes to optimizing the response to psychostimulants used as medical intervention.

The systematic review of Händel et al. was centered around assessing the contribution of using polyunsaturated fatty acids (PUFAs, concretely omega 3 and omega 6) in the treatment plans of ADHD children and adolescents, obtained from randomized clinical trials [9]. Based on a substantial body of evidence, this review concluded that the benefits of PUFAs were not clear on core symptoms of ADHD reported by parents and teachers, neither were they clear on other behavioral measures nor on quality of life measures. However, the authors' advise that these global results should be considered with caution due to discrepancies regarding their methodologies and assessment tools.

An open trial conducted by Yorgidis and colleagues explored the role of oligoantigenic diet (OD) as a therapeutic tool within ADHD children [10] and observed that the combination of this diet and the subsequent food challenge was efficient to identify individual food sensitivity in connection with ADHD. OD is an individualized type of elimination diet aimed at identifying specific foods that worsen psychopathological symptoms, followed by reintroducing other alternative foods that improve neuropsychological performance. The results observed in the study of Yorgidis are relevant considering that some treatment guidelines on ADHD simply recommend restricted/elimination diets among ADHD children with a history of adverse reactions to specific (groups of) foods without providing alternative dietary plans. The basis of the OD is the identification of high food sensitivity in ADHD children, with the objective of including individualized dietary plans within multimodal therapies. Other current studies have also observed that this is a promising approach for decreasing ADHD symptoms [11,12].

On the other hand, some studies have also assessed the role of caffeine exposure within the ADHD profile and as a therapeutic tool. Since it was observed that both chronic and acute exposure to caffeine impacts the central nervous system modulating neuronal pathways, the possible existence of a link between the modulation of these neurotransmitters and the development/attenuation of neuropsychiatric outcomes is supposed. Animal research has observed that non-toxic doses of caffeine elicit neuro-pharmacological actions by blocking adenosine A receptors in the brain, which leads to the blockade of adenosine kinase and a decrease in the release of adenosine [13]. Since adenosine A2 receptor is a G-protein coupled receptor that regulates several functions in the central nervous system (for example, it is related to dopaminergic functions), it was hypothesized that caffeine could impact the specific symptoms of neurological disorders comprising this neurotransmitter [14]. It could also represent a target for the development of therapeutic plans addressing diverse neuropsychiatric conditions (including ADHD). Within this research area, the study of Vázquet et al. addressed a systematic review of scientific studies focused on the underlying effects of caffeine consumption on treating ADHD-like symptoms in animal studies [15]. The combined results of the 13 selected works suggested the concrete benefit of caffeine treatment, increasing attention levels and improving learning capacity, memory ability and olfactory discrimination without altering blood pressure and body weight. The authors concluded that the cumulate evidence of this review, supported at the neuronal level in animal models, strengthens the hypothesis that the cognitive effects of caffeine could be positive for intervention within ADHD, particularly during adolescence. However, they also observed that some of the reviewed studies provided inconsistent results, particularly concerning data referring to caffeine effects on locomotor activity and impulsivity. Exploring clues to explain the effects of caffeine within ADHD treatment plans is a growing area that warrants further research.

3. Diet Intervention on Anxiety and Depression

Studies have identified a strong link between persistent stress and several adverse effects on the body's immune, neuroendocrine, cardiovascular and central nervous systems [16]. Untreated chronic stress could also lead to other serious mental disorders such as anxiety and depression [17], recognized as the most common psychopathological states with high prevalence in contemporary societies. With an impact rate of around 332 million people for depression and 264 million for anxiety, depression and anxiety are the main reasons for disability worldwide [18]. Unfortunately, their rising prevalence, published globally during the last two years and characterized by COVID-19 [19], has increased awareness surrounding these disorders, recognizing them as major contributors to the global burden of disease.

Medical intervention (benzodiazepines and antidepressants) plus cognitive behavioral therapy is considered the gold standard intervention for depression and anxiety states. However, in some cases, these treatments are not effective, induce severe side effects (mostly medications) or are not recommended due to the patients' characteristics (for example, very young or older age, or high risk of interaction with other medications). This scenario guided the search for new interventions for assisting in the prevention and management of anxiety-depressive illnesses, with less risk of side effects. Since the prerequisite to developing adequate evidence-based clinical guidelines is to assimilate dietary patterns and identify the biological mechanisms of action of critical nutrients [20], studies within the nutritional psychiatry research area have established similar pathophysiology systems related to the onset and development of depression and anxiety. Both mental illnesses increase oxidative stress, heighten inflammatory markers and over-activate stress and neuroplasticity pathways, with the result of altered neurotransmission and other brain structural changes [21,22]. The microbiome–gut–brain axis was identified as a key mediating pathway for the biological processes (including hypothalamic–pituitary–adrenal axis, immune function, modulation of BDNF and serotonin neurotransmission) [23]. Compelling evidence has encouraged research into the complementary use of nutrition supplements plus dietary plans with the aim to impact the pathways implied in psychiatric disorders. Studies have also reported common dietary factors in the underlying processes of anxiety and depression; particularly diets or supplements that are high in antioxidants and anti-inflammatories (such as Vitamin C, Vitamin A, Polyphenol and beta-carotene) have shown an inverse relationship with depression and anxiety severity levels [24,25].

Dietary changes and nutritional supplementation may also be beneficial in improving treatment response and quality of life among patients with depression and anxiety. The comprehensive scoping review conducted by Aucoin and colleagues [26], with a full-text review of 1541 articles selected (comprising animal research, human observational/experimental studies and meta-analyses of randomized trials), observed that decreased anxiety levels were related to healthy nutrition practices. Concretely, the least severe anxiety states reported dietary patterns characterized by caloric restriction, breakfast consumption, a broad spectrum of micronutrients–macronutrients supplementation (such as minerals, trace elements, vitamins, essential fatty acids), use of probiotics and intake of a range of fruits and vegetables. On the other extreme of the anxiety continuum, the most impairing states were associated with a high fat/high sugar/high cholesterol/high trans-fat diet, unbalanced tryptophan and protein and a high intake of carbohydrates. Regarding the prospective studies assessing treatment efficacy for dietary interventions, this scoping study concluded that the elimination of inflammatory foods, nutritional supplements and increases in the intakes of fruits and vegetables could contribute to better therapy responses, but only in combination with exercise and the other psychiatric and psychological interventions.

The meta-analysis of Berthelot and colleagues selecting randomized controlled trials concluded that fasting interventions, compared to control groups, achieved lower anxiety and depression levels, and it was also useful to decrease body mass index levels [27]. The benefit on weight was also interpreted as relevant since overweight and obesity are common among patients with depressive and anxiety states [28], and this comorbid condition is related to poor therapy response. [29]. The treatments meta-analyzed by Berthelot also showed to be safe in patients with other comorbid physical conditions, including type-2 diabetes. However, results did not allow recommending the fasting intervention type according to the baseline profiles (diagnostic subtype and severity).

This set of results are consistent with established evidence regarding healthy eating patterns and improvements in anxiety and depression states and the benefit of complementing the classic treatments with dietary interventions according to the specific needs of each patient. The low cost and the high effectiveness of these complementary plans may also confer additional benefits to physical aspects of health [30].

4. Diet Intervention on the Autism Spectrum

It is known that some mental health conditions, such as those included within the autism spectrum, could severely impact the appetite and food choices [31]. Autism or autistic spectrum disorder (ASD) constitutes a complex wide spectrum of neurodevelopmental conditions typically identified during the first years of life, which affects brain functions and particularly areas of communication skills and social interaction. Typical symptoms are poor eye contact, refusing to be held or cuddled, impaired talking capacities, repeated–compulsive behaviors, restricted interests, lack of enthusiasm in playing with other children and lack of imaginative play. These impairments affect eating habits, encompassing some unhealthy concerns [32]: (a) eating an inadequate amount of food (some children within the ASD spectrum may show difficulties focusing on one concrete taste for an extended time or for eating a complete meal); (b) high sensitivity to the taste, smell, color or texture of foods, companied with avoiding specific foods or whole food groups (ASD individuals may express strong food dislikes and limited food selection); (c) potential medication interactions, which can lower appetite and/or even affect the absorption of certain elements (such as minerals and vitamins); and (d) the tendency of some ASD individuals to decrease their food intake as the children move from infancy to toddlerhood and childhood. Other frequent behavioral problems related to eating are gorging/hoarding food in the mouth, gagging/vomiting due to unliked food, not wanting to sit for meals or refusing social eating habits, sniffing/inspecting their own and others' foods and taking food from others' plates.

A current empirical study aimed to explore the dietary patterns and nutrient intakes of ASD children compared to a healthy control group [33] observed that the autism group was characterized by higher consumption of cereals and pasta and a smaller intake of lean meat and eggs compared to reference dietary guidelines. The consumption of fruit, vegetables and fish was similar between the groups (lower than expected for a balanced diet), while the amounts of fatty meat and derivates, snacks, sweets and baked goods confectionery was higher than expected in an adequate diet in both ASD patients and controls. This research also observed that less than one-half of the ASD children tolerated solid foods and that compared to the control group, nutrient intakes were higher for energy, fat and saturated fat and lower for fiber, iron, iodine and some vitamins. These results are consistent with other studies identifying inadequate micronutrient intakes for some minerals among individuals within the autistic spectrum [34]. These individuals could benefit from adequate monitoring of nutritional presence and, if necessary, introducing supplements into their diet [35].

However, most interventions used to treat dysfunctional eating behaviors within the ASD spectrum (such as escape extinction, fading techniques and positive reinforcement) are aimed to increase the volume of food consumed, and few consider increasing the variety of foods and addressing protein–energy–micronutrient deficiencies [36,37]. Other dietary restrictions imposed by parents/caretakers as a therapeutic tool aimed to improve behavior and gastrointestinal symptoms (such as gluten-free or casein-free diets) further intensify the dietary vulnerability of individuals with ASD and in turn, could represent a big barrier to balanced eating [38,39]. Because nutritional status is the consequence of complex mechanisms and interactions, and since micronutrient deficiencies can seriously interact with development (such as scurvy due to low vitamin intake or reduced bone growth due to low levels of calcium), it is essential to explore the effectiveness of multi-component interventions aimed to provide more balanced eating within ASD [40].

5. Conclusions

Problems related to nutrition are often overlooked in patients with common mental health disorders (such as depression, anxiety, ADHD and ASD) towards interventions focused on medication complemented by behavior/psychotherapy treatments. Current research within the nutritional psychiatry area provides evidence regarding the role of nutrition and diet on these psychiatric conditions and offers a basis for developing new evidence-based intervention plans from a multidisciplinary perspective. Given the multifaceted and complex nature of mental and neurodevelopmental problems, the onset at early ages of the child (particularly for ADHD and ASD) and its persistent presentation across development stages (from early childhood to older age), the findings of these works could also contribute to the elaboration of guidelines/recommendations for improving the caring capacity of healthcare practitioners and family caregivers. In the end, improving the nutritional status of the patient will contribute to the individuals' wellbeing and facilitate better progression of medical conditions.

However, the design of effective dietary plans is based on the existence of reliable and valid assessment tools. Unfortunately, the current evidence does not propose nutritional assessment instruments specifically developed for individuals with different mental disorders (such as depression, anxiety, ADHD and ASD). Nutritional psychiatric research warrants additional attention and effort, combining varied methodologies and analyzing larger groups (clinical and population-based samples). Therefore, based on the existing research, dietary markers (foods variety, nutrients intake, sensory issues, preferences/restrictions and dietary intakes), biochemical indexes (vitamins, proteins, minerals, carbohydrates, lipids and other essential nutrients) and anthropometric evaluation (length-for-age, weight-for-age, weight-for-length, head circumference and other age-related-developmental indexes) should be key components of these measurement tools.

As a final thought, the study of how nutrition and mental health are linked is a growing research area, and the results obtained so far are highly promising. The ultimate objective is to facilitate new strategies for improving the quality of life and health of people with mental illness and to prevent the onset, aggravation and negative impacts of diseases.

Funding: This research received no external funding.

Data Availability Statement: No original data has been analyzed for this manuscript.

Acknowledgments: This manuscript was supported by the Catalan Institution for Research and Advanced Studies (ICREA-Academia, 2021-Programme). This funding institution had no role in the writing of the manuscript, or the decision to submit the paper for publication.

Conflicts of Interest: The authors declare no conflict of interest.

References

1. World Health Organization. *Nutrition, Overweight and Obesity*; World Health Organization: Geneva, Switzerland, 2021. Available online: https://www.euro.who.int/en/health-topics/disease-prevention/nutrition/publications/2021/fact-sheet-on-the-sdgs-nutrition,-overweight-and-obesity-2021 (accessed on 24 December 2021).
2. World Health Organization. *Thirteenth General Programme of Work, 2019–2023*; World Health Organization: Geneva, Switzerland, 2018. Available online: https://www.who.int/about/what-we-do/thirteenth-general-programme-of-work-2019---2023 (accessed on 24 December 2021).
3. World Health Organization. *Healthy Diet*; World Health Organization: Geneva, Switzerland, 2020. Available online: https://www.who.int/news-room/fact-sheets/detail/healthy-diet (accessed on 24 December 2021).
4. Polanczyk, G.V.; Willcutt, E.G.; Salum, G.A.; Kieling, C.; Rohde, L.A. ADHD prevalence estimates across three decades: An updated systematic review and meta-regression analysis. *Int. J. Epidemiol.* **2014**, *43*, 434–442. [CrossRef] [PubMed]
5. Di Lorenzo, R.; Balducci, J.; Poppi, C.; Arcolin, E.; Cutino, A.; Ferri, P.; D'Amico, R.; Filippini, T. Children and adolescents with ADHD followed up to adulthood: A systematic review of long-term outcomes. *Acta Neuropsychiatr.* **2021**, *33*, 283–298. [CrossRef] [PubMed]
6. Dalsgaard, S.; Østergaard, S.D.; Leckman, J.F.; Mortensen, P.B.; Pedersen, M.G. Mortality in children, adolescents, and adults with attention deficit hyperactivity disorder: A nationwide cohort study. *Lancet* **2015**, *385*, 2190–2196. [CrossRef]
7. Pelsser, L.M.; Frankena, K.; Toorman, J.; Rodrigues Pereira, R. Diet and ADHD, Reviewing the Evidence: A Systematic Review of Meta-Analyses of Double-Blind Placebo-Controlled Trials Evaluating the Efficacy of Diet Interventions on the Behavior of Children with ADHD. *PLoS ONE* **2017**, *12*, e0169277. [CrossRef] [PubMed]
8. Granero, R.; Pardo-Garrido, A.; Carpio-Toro, I.L.; Ramírez-Coronel, A.A.; Martínez-Suárez, P.C.; Reivan-Ortiz, G.G. The Role of Iron and Zinc in the Treatment of ADHD among Children and Adolescents: A Systematic Review of Randomized Clinical Trials. *Nutrients* **2021**, *13*, 4059. [CrossRef] [PubMed]
9. Händel, M.N.; Rohde, J.F.; Rimestad, M.L.; Bandak, E.; Birkefoss, K.; Tendal, B.; Lemcke, S.; Callesen, H.E. Efficacy and Safety of Polyunsaturated Fatty Acids Supplementation in the Treatment of Attention Deficit Hyperactivity Disorder (ADHD) in Children and Adolescents: A Systematic Review and Meta-Analysis of Clinical Trials. *Nutrients* **2021**, *13*, 1226. [CrossRef] [PubMed]
10. Yorgidis, E.; Beiner, L.; Blazynski, N.; Schneider-Momm, K.; Clement, H.-W.; Rauh, R.; Schulz, E.; Clement, C.; Fleischhaker, C. Individual Behavioral Reactions in the Context of Food Sensitivities in Children with Attention-Deficit/Hyperactivity Disorder before and after an Oligoantigenic Diet. *Nutrients* **2021**, *13*, 2598. [CrossRef]
11. Dölp, A.; Schneider-Momm, K.; Heiser, P.; Clement, C.; Rauh, R.; Clement, H.-W.; Schulz, E.; Fleischhaker, C. Oligoantigenic Diet Improves Children's ADHD Rating Scale Scores Reliably in Added Video-Rating. *Front. Psychiatry* **2020**, *11*, e730. [CrossRef]
12. Ly, V.; Bottelier, M.; Hoekstra, P.J.; Arias Vasquez, A.; Buitelaar, J.K.; Rommelse, N.N. Elimination diets' efficacy and mechanisms in attention deficit hyperactivity disorder and autism spectrum disorder. *Eur. Child Adolesc. Psychiatry* **2017**, *26*, 1067–1079. [CrossRef] [PubMed]
13. Alasmari, F. Caffeine induces neurobehavioral effects through modulating neurotransmitters. *Saudi Pharm. J.* **2020**, *28*, 445–451. [CrossRef]
14. Domenici, M.R.; Ferrante, A.; Martire, A.; Chiodi, V.; Pepponi, R.; Tebano, M.T.; Popoli, P. Adenosine A2A receptor as potential therapeutic target in neuropsychiatric disorders. *Pharmacol. Res.* **2019**, *147*, e104338. [CrossRef] [PubMed]
15. Vázquez, J.C.; de la Torre, O.M.; López-Palomé, J.; Redolar-Ripoll, D. Effects of caffeine consumption on Attention Deficit Hyperactivity Disorder (ADHD) treatment: A systematic review of animal studies. *Nutrients* **2022**, in press.
16. Noushad, S.; Ahmed, S.; Ansari, B.; Mustafa, U.H.; Saleem, Y.; Hazrat, H. Physiological biomarkers of chronic stress: A systematic review. *Int. J. Health Sci.* **2021**, *15*, 46–59.
17. Khan, S.; Khan, R.A. Chronic Stress Leads to Anxiety and Depression. *Ann. Psychiatry Ment. Health* **2017**, *5*, e1091. Available online: https://www.jscimedcentral.com/Psychiatry/psychiatry-5-1091.pdf (accessed on 24 December 2021).
18. World Health Organization. *Depression and Other Common Mental Disorders*; World Health Organization: Geneva, Switzerland, 2017. Available online: https://www.who.int/publications/i/item/depression-global-health-estimates (accessed on 24 December 2021).

19. Dragioti, E.; Li, H.; Tsitsas, G.; Lee, K.H.; Choi, J.; Kim, J.; Choi, Y.J.; Tsamakis, K.; Estradé, A.; Agorastos, A.; et al. A large scale meta-analytic atlas of mental health problems prevalence during the COVID-19 early pandemic. *J. Med. Virol.* **2021**, e27549. [CrossRef] [PubMed]
20. Felger, J.C. Imaging the role of inflammation in mood and anxiety-related disorders. *Curr. Neuropharmacol.* **2018**, *16*, 533–558. [CrossRef] [PubMed]
21. Kris-Etherton, P.M.; Petersen, K.S.; Hibbeln, J.R.; Hurley, D.; Kolick, V.; Peoples, S.; Rodriguez, N.; Woodward-Lopez, G. Nutrition and behavioral health disorders: Depression and anxiety. *Nutr. Rev.* **2021**, *79*, 247–260. [CrossRef]
22. Lee, C.-H.; Giuliani, F. The role of inflammation in depression and fatigue. *Front. Immunol.* **2019**, *10*, e1696. [CrossRef] [PubMed]
23. Pereira, G.A.; da Silva, A.; Hermsdorff, H.; Moreira, A.; de Aguiar, A.S. Association of dietary total antioxidant capacity with depression, anxiety, and sleep disorders: A systematic review of observational studies. *J. Clin. Transl. Res.* **2021**, *7*, 631–640. [PubMed]
24. Marx, W.; Moseley, G.; Berk, M.; Jacka, F. Nutritional psychiatry: The present state of the evidence. *Proc. Nutr. Soc.* **2017**, *76*, 427–436. [CrossRef] [PubMed]
25. Lin, K.; Li, Y.; Toit, E.D.; Wendt, L.; Sun, J. Effects of Polyphenol Supplementations on Improving Depression, Anxiety, and Quality of Life in Patients With Depression. *Front. Psychiatry* **2021**, *12*, e765485. [CrossRef] [PubMed]
26. Aucoin, M.; LaChance, L.; Naidoo, U.; Remy, D.; Shekdar, T.; Sayar, N.; Cardozo, V.; Rawana, T.; Chan, I.; Cooley, K. Diet and Anxiety: A Scoping Review. *Nutrients* **2021**, *13*, 4418. [CrossRef] [PubMed]
27. Berthelot, E.; Etchecopar-Etchart, D.; Thellier, D.; Lancon, C.; Boyer, L.; Fond, G. Fasting Interventions for Stress, Anxiety and Depressive Symptoms: A Systematic Review and Meta-Analysis. *Nutrients* **2021**, *13*, 3947. [CrossRef] [PubMed]
28. Silva, D.A.; Coutinho, E.D.S.F.; Ferriani, L.O.; Viana, M.C. Depression subtypes and obesity in adults: A systematic review and meta-analysis. *Obes. Rev.* **2020**, *21*, e12966. [CrossRef] [PubMed]
29. Grigolon, R.B.; Trevizol, A.P.; Gerchman, F.; Bambokian, A.D.; Magee, T.; McIntyre, R.S.; Gomes, F.A.; Brietzke, E.; Mansur, R.B. Is Obesity A Determinant Of Success With Pharmacological Treatment For Depression? A Systematic Review, Meta-Analysis And Meta-Regression. *J. Affect. Disord.* **2021**, *287*, 54–68. [CrossRef]
30. Chatterton, M.L.; Mihalopoulos, C.; O'Neil, A.; Itsiopoulos, C.; Opie, R.; Castle, D.; Dash, S.; Brazionis, L.; Berk, M.; Jacka, F. Economic evaluation of a dietary intervention for adults with major depression (the "SMILES" trial). *BMC Public Health* **2018**, *18*, e599. [CrossRef] [PubMed]
31. Chawner, L.R.; Blundell-Birtill, P.; Hetherington, M.M. Interventions for Increasing Acceptance of New Foods Among Children and Adults with Developmental Disorders: A Systematic Review. *J. Autism Dev. Disord.* **2019**, *49*, 3504–3525. [CrossRef] [PubMed]
32. Margari, L.; Marzulli, L.; Gabellone, A.; de Giambattista, C. Eating and Mealtime Behaviors in Patients with Autism Spectrum Disorder: Current Perspectives. *Neuropsychiatr. Dis. Treat.* **2020**, *16*, 2083–2102. [CrossRef] [PubMed]
33. Plaza-Diaz, J.; Flores-Rojas, K.; Torre-Aguilar, M.J.d.l.; Gomez-Fernández, A.R.; Martín-Borreguero, P.; Perez-Navero, J.L.; Gil, A.; Gil-Campos, M. Dietary Patterns, Eating Behavior, and Nutrient Intakes of Spanish Preschool Children with Autism Spectrum Disorders. *Nutrients* **2021**, *13*, 3551. [CrossRef]
34. Esteban-Figuerola, P.; Canals, J.; Fernandez-Cao, J.C.; Arija Val, V. Differences in food consumption and nutritional intake between children with autism spectrum disorders and typically developing children: A meta-analysis. *Autism* **2019**, *23*, 1079–1095. [CrossRef] [PubMed]
35. Brzoska, A.; Kazek, B.; Koziol, K.; Kapinos-Gorczyca, A.; Ferlewicz, M.; Babraj, A.; Makosz-Raczek, A.; Likus, W.; Paprocka, J.; Matusik, P. Eating Behaviors of Children with Autism-Pilot Study. *Nutrients* **2021**, *13*, 2687. [CrossRef] [PubMed]
36. Ledford, J.R.; Whiteside, E.; Severini, K.E. A systematic review of interventions for feeding-related behaviors for individuals with autism spectrum disorders. *Res. Autism Spectr. Disord.* **2018**, *52*, 69–80. [CrossRef]
37. Tachibana, Y.; Miyazaki, C.; Ota, E.; Mori, R.; Hwang, Y.; Kobayashi, E.; Terasaka, A.; Tang, J.; Kamio, Y. A systematic review and meta-analysis of comprehensive interventions for pre-school children with autism spectrum disorder (ASD). *PLoS ONE* **2017**, *12*, e0186502. [CrossRef] [PubMed]
38. Sathe, N.; Andrews, J.C.; McPheeters, M.L.; Warren, Z.E. Nutritional and Dietary Interventions for Autism Spectrum Disorder: A Systematic Review. *Pediatrics* **2017**, *139*, e20170346. [CrossRef] [PubMed]
39. Alamri, E.S. Efficacy of gluten-and casein-free diets on autism spectrum disorders in children. *Saudi Med. J.* **2020**, *41*, 1041–1046. [CrossRef] [PubMed]
40. Babinska, K.; Celusakova, H.; Belica, I.; Szapuova, Z.; Waczulikova, I.; Nemcsicova, D.; Tomova, A.; Ostatnikova, D. Gastrointestinal Symptoms and Feeding Problems and Their Associations with Dietary Interventions, Food Supplement Use, and Behavioral Characteristics in a Sample of Children and Adolescents with Autism Spectrum Disorders. *Int. J. Environ. Res. Public Health* **2020**, *17*, 6372. [CrossRef]

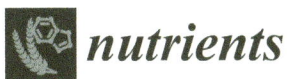

Article

Fasting Interventions for Stress, Anxiety and Depressive Symptoms: A Systematic Review and Meta-Analysis

Elisa Berthelot [1,2], Damien Etchecopar-Etchart [1,2], Dimitri Thellier [3], Christophe Lancon [1,2], Laurent Boyer [1,2] and Guillaume Fond [1,2,*]

[1] Assistance Publique-Hôpitaux de Marseille, Aix-Marseille University, Faculté de Médecine—Secteur Timone, EA 3279: CEReSS—Centre d'Etude et de Recherche sur les Services de Santé et la Qualité de vie, 27 Boulevard Jean Moulin, 13005 Marseille, France; elisa.berthelot@ap-hm.fr (E.B.); damien.etche@gmail.com (D.E.-E.); christophe.lancon@ap-hm.fr (C.L.); laurent.boyer@ap-hm.fr (L.B.)
[2] Fondation Fonda Mental, 94000 Créteil, France
[3] Institut de Neuro-Épidémiologie Tropicale, Université de Limoges, 27 Boulevard Jean Moulin, 13005 Marseille, France; dthellier@icloud.com
* Correspondence: guillaume.fond@gmail.com

Abstract: Background. Fasting interventions have shown effectiveness in alleviating stress, anxiety and depressive symptoms. However, no quantitative analysis has been carried out thus far. The objective was to determine the effectiveness of fasting interventions on stress, anxiety and depression and if these interventions were associated with increased or decreased fatigue/energy. Methods. Overall, 11 studies and 1436 participants were included in the quantitative analyses. Results. After limiting analyses to randomized controlled trials with low risk of bias, we found that fasting groups had lower anxiety (b = −0.508, $p = 0.038$), depression levels (b= −0.281, $p = 0.012$) and body mass index compared to controls without increased fatigue. There was no publication bias and no heterogeneity for these results. These interventions were safe, even in patients with type 2 diabetes. Conclusions. These results should be taken with a caveat. These results are preliminary and encouraging and fasting appears to be a safe intervention. Data are not sufficient to recommend one fasting intervention more than the others. No study was carried out in psychiatric populations and further trials should be carried out in these populations that may be good candidates for fasting interventions.

Keywords: public health; mental health; fasting; antidepressant; depression; anxiety; schizophrenia; physical health; obesity

1. Introduction

Depressive and anxiety disorders are leading worldwide causes of disability and loss of quality-adjusted life year in people aged < 40 years [1]. Antidepressants are the gold standard treatments for these disorders but are effective in only approximately half of the patients and induce frequent side effects. Identifying new pathophysiological pathways to develop personalized treatments for these disorders and improve the benefit/risk ratio is a major challenge of current research. Among these new pathways, the gut–brain axis has generated a lot of interest with the recent discoveries concerning the microbiota and its role in anxiety and depression [2,3]. The field of psychonutrition has developed in parallel with the discovery of the protective role of a healthy/anti-inflammatory diet on depression onset [4,5] and the effectiveness, among other nutrients, of omega 3 fatty acids in the treatment of anxiety and depression [6].

In the 1990s and 2000s, some trials explored the effect of therapeutic fasting (or very low-caloric fasting) on depression and anxiety with inconsistent results and without non-fasting group control [7–9]. Fasting interventions are becoming in parallel more and more popular in the general population. Individuals experiencing these fasts mostly report a subjective psychological improvement.

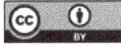

Intermittent fasting is defined by reducing the daily duration of diet intake. Intermittent fasting can take different forms, from fasting one or two days a week to fasting 12 to 18 h a day. The potential effectiveness of intermittent fasting on mood has raised growing interest. Overweight/obesity is associated with increased depression and fasting may be effective in improving depressive symptoms by favoring weight loss [10–13]. In addition to weight loss, rodent and human studies have shown that daily intermittent fasting may switch glucose metabolism to ketone metabolism, inducing anti-inflammatory, anti-oxidative and stress resistance effects [14]. Fasting may improve microbiota disturbances and intestinal inflammation through decreased inflammatory foods intake and decreased blood flow dedicated to digestion [15]. The safety and acceptability of intermittent fasting may be limitations to the development of fasting interventions. Among them, it is unclear if fasting interventions may decrease energy/increase fatigue. This question is of importance as fatigue is a common depressive symptom [16]. Another remaining question is that intermittent fasting is often combined with caloric restriction, and there is a debate to know which is the true effective intervention to improve anxiety and depressive symptoms. To address this question, a randomized controlled trial has been carried out comparing caloric restriction with or without 14 h of restricted feeding in type 2 diabetes patients [17]. The authors concluded that both regimens were associated with improved depression, suggesting that caloric restriction should also be studied among fasting interventions.

The primary objective of this systematic review and meta-analysis was to determine the effectiveness of fasting interventions on stress, anxiety and depression. The secondary objective was to confirm that these interventions were also effective in reducing body mass index and if these interventions were associated with increased or decreased fatigue/energy.

2. Materials and Methods

2.1. Literature Search Strategy

This meta-analysis was conducted in accordance with the Preferred Reporting Items for Systematic reviews and Meta-Analysis guidelines. Systematic bibliographic searches were carried out according to the Cochrane methodology. This project was registered in PROSPERO (reference number CRD42020197359) (https://www.crd.york.ac.uk/prospero/ accessed on 18 August 2020). The search paradigm was based on the PubMed interface (Medline database) and adapted for 2 databases: ScienceDirect and Google Scholar. There were no restrictions for languages and dates. The search paradigm was based on the following combination of MeSH terms "fasting" AND each MeSH terms: "anxiety" OR "stress" OR "mood disorder" OR "depression" OR "depressive". In the case of missing data, authors were contacted by email if possible. The reference lists and bibliographies of relevant reviews and articles retrieved from the database searches were manually searched for additional eligible articles. The last search was carried out on 30 August 2021.

2.2. Eligibility

The inclusion criteria were: (1) any language and date of publication; (2) original research papers; (3) fasting intervention; (4) evaluation of stress and/or anxiety symptoms and/or depression after one fasting intervention with a validated scale; (5) observational studies or controlled trials. The exclusion criterion was diet interventions not directly targeting fasting or caloric restriction. The titles and abstracts were screened by 2 researchers (E.B. and G.F). The full texts of the manuscripts were then reviewed to determine whether a study would be included (E.B. and G.F). In the case of non-consensus, a third author (L.B.) had the final decision for inclusion.

2.3. Data Extraction

Two researchers (E.B. and G.F.) extracted data from the included studies in a systematic manner using a predesigned extraction form. Each discrepancy in data extraction was examined by three authors (E.B, D.E.E and G.F) to reach consensus.

The variables were extracted as follows: study ID and design, author, year, type of study, sample size, fasting intervention description, fasting duration, religious fasting (y/n), fasting intervention including caloric restriction (y/n), socio-demographic data (country, mean age, percentage of men, study including clinical population vs. healthy volunteers, baseline and post-intervention body mass index (mean/standard deviation (SD)), baseline and post-intervention stress, anxiety and depressive symptoms scores in fasting and control groups (mean (SD)), delay between the end of fasting intervention and first evaluation (weeks), and number and type of potential adverse event.

2.4. Study Quality

The study quality was assessed by DEE and GF with the study quality assessment tool for observational cohort or cross-sectional studies for Ramadan studies and for quality assessment tools for controlled studies for fasting intervention controlled trials [18]. In cases of non-consensus, a third author (L.B.) made the final decision for study quality.

2.5. Statistical Analyses

As Ramadan studies were all observational except one [19], we calculated a pre/post Ramadan effect. For controlled trials, we calculated mean standardized estimate between groups receiving fasting intervention vs. controls at the endpoint following the end of fasting intervention (i.e., differential changes from baseline to post-fast in the fasting versus control groups). Heterogeneity between studies was measured by Cochrane's Q test. Publication bias was assessed using Egger's test funnel plot. We used comprehensive meta-analysis software (v3.0), Biostat, Englewood, NJ 07631, USA.

2.6. Role of the Funding Source

This work received no funding. No drug manufacturing company was involved in the study design, the data collection, the data analysis, the data interpretation, the writing of the report, or the decision to submit the report for publication.

3. Results

3.1. Characteristics of Studies

Overall, 11 studies were included [17,19–28] (flow chart, Figure 1). Among the 1436 participants, 1009 subjects experienced Ramadan fasting, 239 received other fasting interventions (2 days/week ($N = 28$) or one day/week fasting ($N = 22$), 14 h restricted fasting with caloric restriction ($N = 27$) or caloric restriction without intermittent fasting (25% caloric restriction or 800 cal/day) ($N = 162$)). One study was included in both Ramadan and fasting controlled studies [19]. Three very low-calorie diet interventions could not be included because both groups received fasting interventions [7–9].

3.2. Ramadan Studies

Ramadan study (Figure 2) characteristics are presented in Table 1 and study quality in Supplementary Table S1. Overall, five studies (1009 participants) [19,22,23,26,28] were included in the Ramadan studies. Two studies were carried out in Iran [22,23], one in Germany [19], one in Turkey [26], and one in Kuwait [28]. One study [22] was carried out in hospital nurses, one in a type II diabetes mellitus population [28], and the others in healthy volunteers [23].

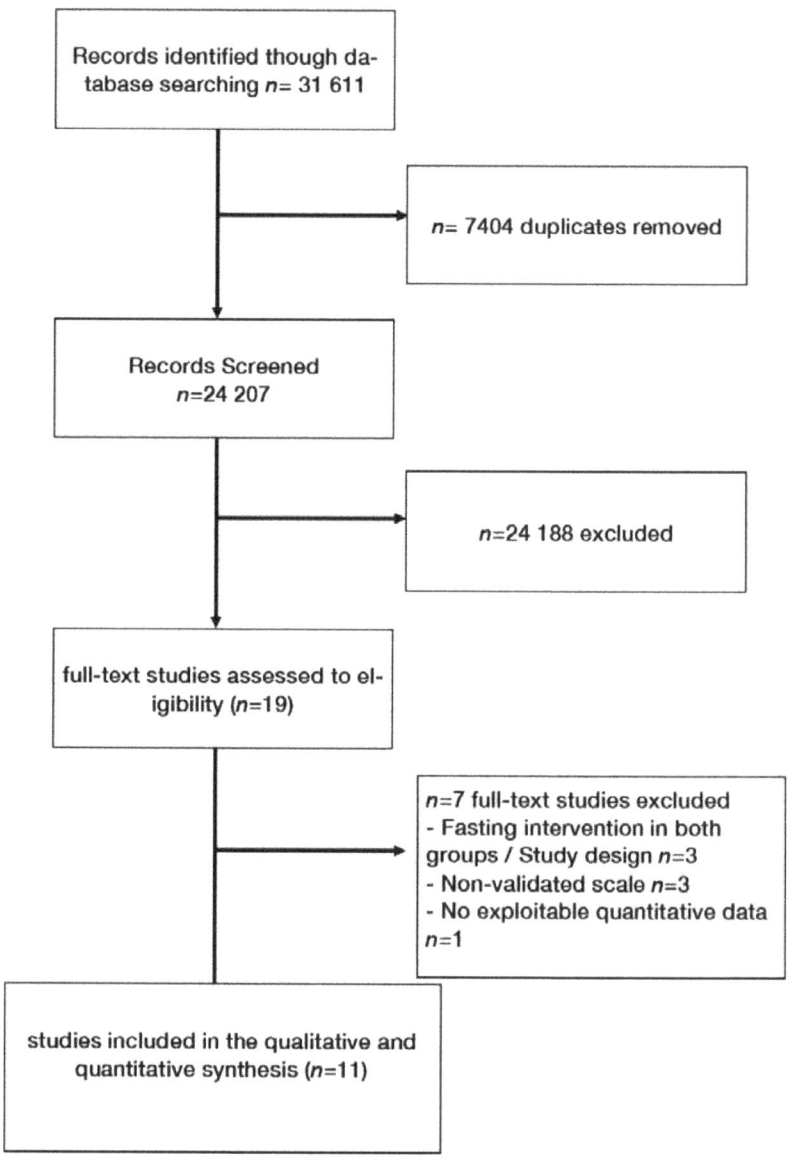

Figure 1. Flow chart.

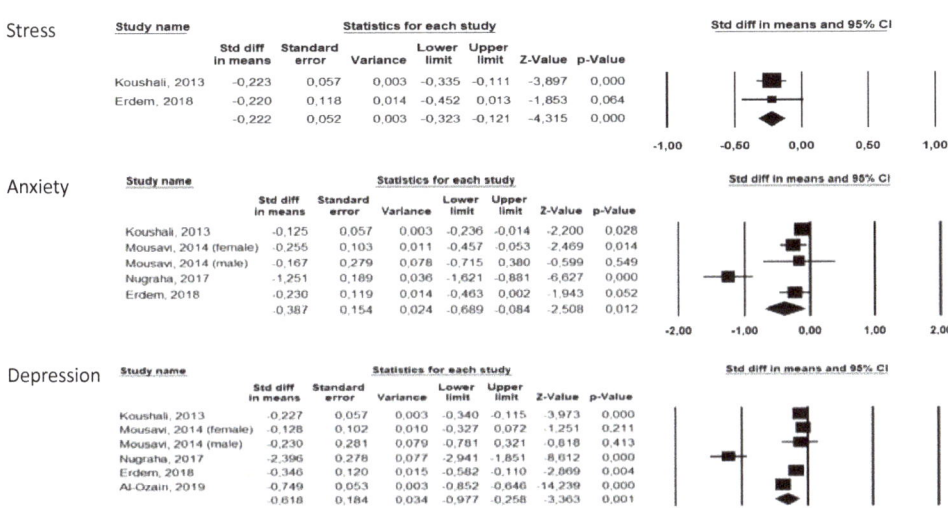

Figure 2. Forests plots of Ramadan studies for stress, anxiety and depression.

Overall, Ramadan was associated with improved stress (b = −0.222 [−0.323;−0.121], $p < 0.0001$, I2 = 0), improved anxiety (b = −0.387 [−0.689;−0.084], $p = 0.012$, I2 = 87.79) and improved depression (b = −0.618 [−0.977;−0.258], $p = 0.001$, I2 = 95.32).

Four studies were classified with moderate risk of bias [19,23,26,28] and one with high risk of bias [22] (Supplementary Table S1). Removing this study did not change our results. The moderate risk of bias was due to studies using self-reported questionnaires and participants being aware of the exposure, as for all nutritional intervention studies.

Funnel plots for Ramadan studies are presented in Supplementary Figure S1. We found no publication bias (Egger's tests > 0.05 for anxiety and depression).

The observational Ramadan studies did not report fasting's adverse events [22,23,26,28]. Fatigue was reported only in the controlled study [19]. Ramadan was associated with increased fatigue during the first week but decreased fatigue during week 2 to 4 and decreased sleepiness during the whole of Ramadan. No study reported dropout due to inability to follow Ramadan.

3.3. Fasting Controlled Trials

Fasting controlled trials (Figure 3) characteristics are presented in Table 1 and study quality in Supplementary Table S2. Seven studies (452 participants, 264 receiving fasting intervention, 188 being controls) were included (five randomized controlled trials [17,20,21,24,25] and two controlled trials [19,27]). The two studies carried out in Malaysia assessed the effectiveness of a 12-week, 300–500 kCal daily caloric restriction associated with 2 days a week of Sunnah Muslim fasting [20,21]. One study carried out in the Czech Republic studied the effects of 12 weeks of caloric restriction with or without 14 h/day intermittent fasting in a diabetes population [17]. One US study measured the effects of 104 weeks of 25% caloric restriction [24]. Among the three studies carried out in Germany, one studied the effects of Ramadan [19], one the effects of 12 weeks of an 800 Cal/day low calorie diet [25] and one the effects of 8 weeks of one day per week fasting, totaling 24 h a week [27].

Table 1. Study characteristics.

Study	Country	N	N F	N C	N(%) Men	Design	Population	Fasting Intervention	Controls	Endpoint *	Scales **	Authors' Conclusion	Adverse Events	N Dropout Fasting	N Dropout Controls
Koushali (2013) [22]	Iran	313	313	NA	177(56.5%)	OBS	Hospital nurses	Ramadan	NA	1 to 2	Anxiety: DASS21 Depression: DASS21	Depression and stress were significantly reduced ($p < 0.05$) but not anxiety.	md	NA	NA
Mousavi (2014) [3]	Iran	110	110	NA	13(11.8%)	OBS	Residents of Kermanshah city	Ramadan	NA	MD	Anxiety: GHQ subscore Depression: GHQ subscore Stress: GHQ	Significant reduction in anxiety ($p = 0.011$) but no significant reduction in depression ($p > 0.05$) after Ramadan.	md	NA	NA
Erdem (2018) [6]	Turkey	73	73	NA	63(86.3%)	OBS	Muslim healthy volunteers	Ramadan	NA	0	Anxiety: DASS42 Anxiety: DASS anxiety Depression: DASS	Significant reduction in depression ($p = 0.001$), anxiety ($p = 0.01$) and stress ($p = 0.002$) scores after Ramadan.	md	NA	NA
Al-Ozairi (2019) [8]	Kuwait	463	463	NA	251(54.2%)	OBS	Type 2 diabetes Muslim patients ≥21 years	Ramadan	NA	4-6	Depression: PHQ-9	Significant reduction in depressive symptoms after Ramadan ($p < 0.05$).	md	NA	NA
Nugraha (2017) [19]	Germany	50	25	25	50(100%)	CT	Healthy male volunteers ≥ 18 years (mostly students)	Ramadan	No fasting and no other intervention	1	Anxiety: HADS Depression: BDI-II	Significant reduction in depressive symptoms after Ramadan ($p < 0.05$).	Increased fatigue during first week of Ramadan, then decreased fatigue during week 2 to 4 but decreased sleepiness during whole Ramadan.	3/28(10.7%) (2 time schedule, 1 other reason)	2/28(7.6%) (other reason)
Teng (2011) [20]	Malaysia	25	12	13	25(100%)	CT	Healthy men aged 50 to 70 years, BMI 23.0 to 29.9 kg/m^2	Reduction in 300 to 500 kcal/day from thei habitual energy intake + two days of Muslim sunnah* fasting per week 12 weeks	No fasting and no other intervention	0	Depression: BDI-II	Non-significant reduction in depressive symptoms after fasting intervention ($p > 0.05$).	Adverse events were not reported but 2 participants were unable to follow the fasting intervention	2/14(14.2%) (unable to follow the fasting intervention)	1/14(7.1%) (personal reasons)

Table 1. *Cont.*

Study	Country	N	N F	N C	N(%) Men	Design	Population	Fasting Intervention	Controls	Endpoint *	Scales **	Authors' Conclusion	Adverse Events	N Dropout Fasting	N Dropout Controls
Hussin (2013) [31]	Malaysia	32	16	16	32(100%)	RCT	Healthy men aged 50 to 70 years, BMI 23.0 to 29.9 kg/m²	Reduction of 300 to 500 kcal/day from their habitual energy intake + two days of Muslim sunnah * fasting per week 12 weeks	No fasting and no other intervention	0	Depression: BDI-II Fatigue: POMS	Non-significant reduction in depressive symptoms after fasting intervention ($p > 0.05$).	No reported adverse events.	0(0%)	1/16(6.2%)
Kahleova (2015) [17]	Czech Republic	54	27	27	29(54%)	RCT	Patient with type 2 diabetes, mean age 59.4 years, mean BMI 32.6 kg/m²	Time Restricted feeding (14 h fasting/day) + caloric restriction 12 weeks	6 meals/day (3 meals + 3 snacks)	0	Depression: BDI-II	Significant reduction in depression score was decreased in the fasting group ($p < 0.05$), and feelings of hunger were greater than in the control group. Quality of life increased ($p < 0.01$) comparably under both regimens.	No reported adverse events.	3/27(11.1%) (1 personal reasons, 2 lack of motivation)	4/27(14.8%) (2 personal reasons, 2 lack of motivation)
Martin(2016) [24]	USA	218	143	75	66(30%)	RCT	Healthy men aged 20 to 50 years and women aged 20 to 47 years, with a BMI between 22.0 and 28.0	25% Caloric Restriction 104 weeks	No fasting and no other intervention	0	Depression: BDI-II Fatigue: POMS	Significant improvement in the depression score ($p < 0.05$), tension ($p < 0.01$), and General health ($p < 0.001$).	No reported adverse events but 3/117(2.6%) participants of the fasting group were removed for safety reasons (not detailed).	26/143(18.2%) (8 withdrew consent, 6 moved away from study site, 6 for personal and other reasons, 3 women became pregnant, 3 withdrawn for safety)	5/75(6.7%) (3 women became pregnant, 1 withdrew consent)
Prehn (2017) [25]	Germany	37	19	18	0(0%)	RCT	Older obese women, mean age 61 years, mean BMI 35	Low calorie diet (800 kcal/l) 12 weeks	No fasting and no other intervention	0	Anxiety: STAI Depression: BDI-II	Reduction in Beck's depression score ($p < 0.001$) and anxiety score ($p < 0.004$) in the fasting group.	No reported adverse events but 6 subjects were excluded for instruction failure without details.	5/23(21.7%) (personal reasons)	5/24(20.8%)

Table 1. Cont.

Study	Country	N	N F	N C	N(%) Men	Design	Population	Fasting Intervention	Controls	Endpoint *	Scales **	Authors' Conclusion	Adverse Events	N Dropout Fasting	N Dropout Controls
Kessler (2018) [27]	Germany	36	22	14	14 (39)%	CT	Healthy volunteers	Fixed fasting day per week for 8 weeks, a fixed day 8 weeks	2 groups counseling sessions for healthy diet + waiting list for fasting intervention	0	Anxiety: HADS-A Depression: HADS-D Fatigue: POMS	Significant within-group differences in the fasting group were observed after 6 months for the HADS total score, and the HADS depression and anxiety subscales, the POMS total score (including subscales for positive mood and vigor).	Adverse events: headache, migraine, nausea, ravenousness, circulatory disturbance, hunger, general feeling of weakness, tiredness, stomach ache, meteorism, heartburn, and cold sensations in the body.	N = 4/22 (9.1%) (2 declined to further participate, 2 lost of follow-up)	N = 2/14 (14.2%)

* in weeks after end of fasting intervention. ** all scales were self-reported questionnaires. BDI-II, Beck Depression Inventory. DASS, Depression Anxiety Stress Scale (DASS-42). GHQ, General Health Questionnaire. GHQ-28, General Health Questionnaire-28. HADS, Hospitalization Anxiety and Depression scale. POMS, Profile of Mood states. PHQ, Patient Health Questionnaire. STAI, State-Trait Anxiety Inventory. F, Fasting. C, Controls. MD, missing data. OBS, observational. RCT, randomized controlled trial. SD, standardized deviation. NA: not adapted.

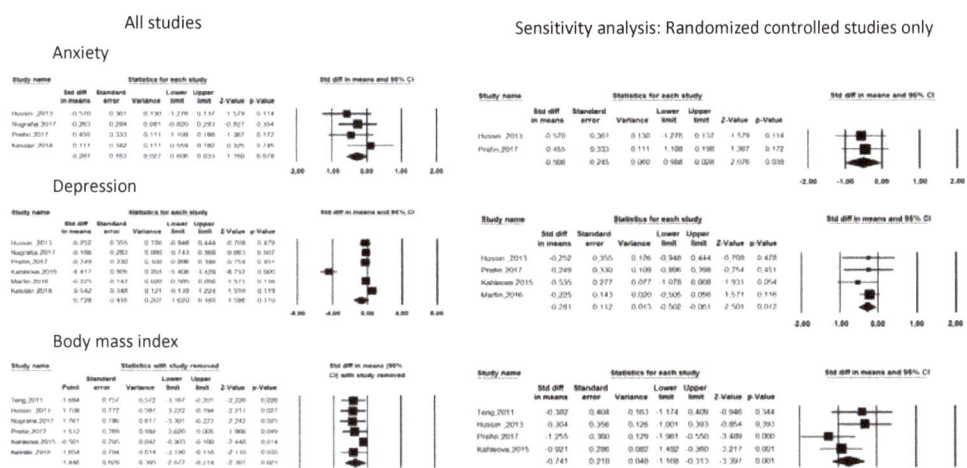

Figure 3. Forest plots of fasting intervention controlled studies for anxiety, depression and body mass index.

Overall, the fasting groups were not found to have lower anxiety or depression levels compared to control groups at the end of fasting ($p > 0.05$, Figure 3), but they were found to have lower body mass index (b = $-1.446[-2.677; -0.274]$, $p = 0.021$).

After removing the two non-randomized controlled trials [19,27], fasting groups were found to have lower anxiety and depression levels (respectively, b = $-0.508[-0.988; -0.028]$, $p = 0.038$, I2 = 0 and b = $-0.281[-0.502; -0.061]$, $p = 0.012$, I2 = 0).

Four randomized controlled trials were evaluated to have low risk of bias [17,20,21,24], one with intermediate risk of bias [25] and the two controlled trials were evaluated to have a high risk of bias [19,27].

There was no publication bias for anxiety and depression (Egger's tests > 0.05) but a publication bias for body mass index (Egger's test = 0.01). Funnel plots are presented in Supplementary Figure S2.

Fatigue was measured in four studies [19,21,24,27]. The fasting groups were not found to have lower or increased fatigue levels at the end of fasting compared to control groups ($p > 0.05$, data not shown). Limiting the analysis to randomized controlled trials [21,24] did not change our results.

Overall, 42 (15.4%) dropouts were reported in fasting groups and 20 (10.2%) in control groups ($p > 0.05$). Among dropouts of fasting interventions, two diabetic patients reported a lack of motivation for 2 meals a day [17], two participants were unable to follow the two days/week fasting combined with caloric restriction for 12 weeks [20] and three participants were removed for safety reasons for 104 weeks of 25% caloric restriction [24]. The other dropouts were for reasons not related to fasting or for unknown reasons.

Only one study reported detailed adverse events for 1 day/week fasting [27]. These adverse events were: headache, migraine, nausea, ravenousness, circulatory disturbance, hunger, general feeling of weakness, tiredness, stomach ache, meteorism, heartburn, and cold sensations in the body.

4. Discussion

In our meta-analysis including 11 studies and 1436 participants, we found that post-Ramadan scores for stress, anxiety and depression were lower compared to those before Ramadan. In fasting controlled trials, we found no significant effect of fasting on anxiety and depression when analyzing all studies. However, we found that fasting groups had lower anxiety and depression levels compared to control groups when limiting the analyses to randomized controlled trials. Fasting was associated with decreased body mass index in all studies without increased fatigue in fasting groups compared to controls. Adverse events were only reported for 1 day/week fasting.

First, we found a positive effect of Ramadan on stress, anxiety and depression. Ramadan is a religious fasting, i.e., including a spiritual and social dimension that may be missing in other forms of fasting. One may hypothesize that depression improvement may not be only due to fasting but also to other lifestyle modifications. For example, Ramadan fasting includes tobacco abstinence, and tobacco abstinence has been associated with improved depressive symptoms [29]. As Ramadan is a dry fasting between sunrise and sunset, the Ramadan fasters may wake up earlier in the morning to feed before sunrise and may therefore reduce their sleep duration. Sleep reduction has been associated with depression improvement [30] and may also play a role in the observed results. Despite its significance, we found heterogeneous results across Ramadan studies for anxiety and depression. We have identified the following factors that may explain this heterogeneity: country/cultural context, clinical (diabetes) vs. non clinical populations, various delay between end of Ramadan and first endpoint evaluation (from 0 to 6 weeks), various scales to assess stress, anxiety and depressive symptoms, various ages and sex ratios. These variables could not be tested due to the small number of studies. Other uncaptured data, such as socioeconomic environment, addictive behaviors, sleep, diet, physical activity and physical comorbidities, including overweight/obesity, may also contribute to heterogeneity. For example, the German study included only healthy male students [19] and the effect of Ramadan on anxiety was much higher in this study compared to the others. However, the results were still significant after removing this study. It should be underlined that all scales to evaluate stress, anxiety or depression were self-reported, and that clinician-rated scales could be useful to confirm these results.

The second major finding is the result of fasting controlled trials. Our overall results were not significant (with a trend toward significance for anxiety, $p = 0.07$). However, after removing two studies with a high risk of bias, the results became significant with low heterogeneity. These results are encouraging to pursue research on fasting intervention effects on mental health, especially in psychiatric samples that have been untested thus far. It should be underlined that the mean stress/anxiety/depression scores were mostly under the pathological rank at baseline, suggesting that fasting interventions are effective for moving from a "healthy" to "even healthier" mood. Despite this fact, the effect sizes indicated a mild effect for depression and moderate effect for anxiety when limited to randomized controlled trials. As most interventions are most effective in patients with more severe baseline symptoms, we believe that fasting interventions should therefore be effective in psychiatric samples. Moreover, we found that patients receiving these interventions benefited from body mass index reduction. Obesity is common in patients with major depression and may influence psychiatric trajectory [31,32]. Intentional weight loss improves the symptoms of depression [10]. However, no study explored if fasting interventions were more effective in overweight participants and it remains to be determined if body mass index is correlated with depressive symptoms. It remains also to be determined if overeating is conversely associated with impaired mood and the direction of the causal relationship [33]. Animal studies also suggest that fasting improves oxidative stress [34]. Further studies should explore if the improvement of oxidative stress parameters would be associated with improved anxiety/depression in humans.

Adverse events were poorly reported. The only study reporting adverse events was those exploring the effects of 24 h/week fasting. Daily intermittent fasting may be effective in limiting these adverse events. The absence of significant dropout rate differences between fasting and control groups is encouraging for the acceptability of fasting interventions. It should be underlined that two meals/day associated with caloric restriction appeared as a safe intervention in patients with diabetes. No hypoglycemia was reported in this study. Metabolic disorders are frequent in psychiatric populations and should therefore not be a limitation to test fasting interventions in psychiatry. Additional data are needed to confirm these preliminary results.

Strengths. We used the most recent meta-analysis standards to carry out the present meta-analysis. A comprehensive search following PRISMA criteria has been carried out, and we used leave-1-out analyses and quality evaluations to determine the risk of bias. The present work therefore adds important knowledge in the field.

Limitations. Our results must be interpreted with caution. Only 11 studies with relatively small sample sizes were included. Four Ramadan studies were observational and two fasting controlled trials were not randomized. The small number of studies did not enable us to carry out sensitivity analyses. An important limitation and direction for future research is that our results were insufficient to determine if caloric restriction is the true effective intervention to improve anxiety or depression, or if intermittent fasting (time-restricted feeding) may have a specific effect. Lastly, although visual inspection of funnel plots did not suggest publication bias, definitive confidence in excluding publication bias was limited by the small number of studies included in our funnel plots. Very low-calorie interventions could not be included in the quantitative analyses. However, most of them reported mood improvement after these interventions. Further trials are therefore warranted to explore their effectiveness.

5. Conclusions

Preliminary evidence suggests that fasting interventions may have a positive effect on anxiety, depression and body mass index reduction without increasing fatigue. It remains unknown if caloric restriction is the true effective component of fasting or if intermittent fasting may increase its effectiveness on stress, anxiety and depressive symptoms. A 12-week intermittent fasting associated with caloric restriction appears as a safe and acceptable intervention, even in patients with diabetes. Further randomized controlled trials are warranted to strengthen these results, especially in psychiatric populations that have not been tested thus far.

Supplementary Materials: The following are available online at https://www.mdpi.com/article/10.3390/nu13113947/s1, Figure S1: Funnel plots of Ramadan studies; Figure S2: Funnel plots of fasting controlled trials; Table S1: Study quality for Ramadan studies, Table S2: Study quality for fasting controlled trials.

Author Contributions: Conceptualization, G.F. and L.B.; methodology, L.B.; software, L.B.; validation, L.B.; formal analysis, L.B.; investigation, E.B. and G.F.; resources, E.B. and G.F.; data curation, G.F.; writing—original draft preparation, E.B. and G.F.; writing—review and editing, D.E.-E., D.T., C.L., G.F. and L.B.; supervision, G.F. and L.B. All authors have read and agreed to the published version of the manuscript.

Funding: This work received no funding. No drug manufacturing company was involved in the study design, the data collection, the data analysis, the data interpretation, the writing of the report, or the decision to submit the report for publication.

Institutional Review Board Statement: Not applicable.

Informed Consent Statement: Not applicable.

Conflicts of Interest: The authors declare no conflict of interest.

References

1. Vos, T.; Lim, S.S.; Abbafati, C.; Abbas, K.M.; Abbasi, M.; Abbasifard, M.; Abbasi-Kangevari, M.; Abbastabar, H.; Abd-Allah, F.; Abdelalim, A.; et al. Global Burden of 369 Diseases and Injuries in 204 Countries and Territories, 1990–2019: A Systematic Analysis for the Global Burden of Disease Study 2019. *Lancet* **2020**, *396*, 1204–1222. [CrossRef]
2. Chevalier, G.; Siopi, E.; Guenin-Macé, L.; Pascal, M.; Laval, T.; Rifflet, A.; Boneca, I.G.; Demangel, C.; Colsch, B.; Pruvost, A.; et al. Effect of gut microbiota on depressive-like behaviors in mice is mediated by the endocannabinoid system. *Nat. Commun.* **2020**, *11*, 1–15. [CrossRef] [PubMed]
3. Fond, G.B.; Lagier, J.-C.; Honore, S.; Lancon, C.; Korchia, T.; De Verville, P.-L.S.; Llorca, P.-M.; Auquier, P.; Guedj, E.; Boyer, L. Microbiota-Orientated Treatments for Major Depression and Schizophrenia. *Nutrients* **2020**, *12*, 1024. [CrossRef]

4. Lassale, C.; Batty, G.; Baghdadli, A.; Jacka, F.; Villegas, A.S.; Kivimäki, M.; Akbaraly, T. Healthy dietary indices and risk of depressive outcomes: A systematic review and meta-analysis of observational studies. *Mol. Psychiatry* **2019**, *24*, 965–986. [CrossRef]
5. Matison, A.P.; Mather, K.A.; Flood, V.M.; Reppermund, S. Associations between nutrition and the incidence of depression in middle-aged and older adults: A systematic review and meta-analysis of prospective observational population-based studies. *Ageing Res. Rev.* **2021**, *70*, 101403. [CrossRef] [PubMed]
6. Liao, Y.; Xie, B.; Zhang, H.; He, Q.; Guo, L.; Subramanieapillai, M.; Fan, B.; Lu, C.; McIntyre, R.S. Efficacy of omega-3 PUFAs in depression: A meta-analysis. *Transl. Psychiatry* **2019**, *9*, 1–9. [CrossRef] [PubMed]
7. Wadden, T.A.; Mason, G.; Foster, G.D.; Stunkard, A.J.; Prange, A.J. Effects of a very low calorie diet on weight, thyroid hormones and mood. *Int. J. Obes.* **1990**, *14*, 249–258.
8. Wing, R.R.; Marcus, M.D.; Blair, E.H.; Burton, L.R. Psychological Responses of Obese Type II Diabetic Subjects to Very-Low-Calorie Diet. *Diabetes Care* **1991**, *14*, 596–599. [CrossRef] [PubMed]
9. Wadden, T.A.; Stunkard, A.J.; Brownell, K.D.; Day, S.C. A comparison of two very-low-calorie diets: Protein-sparing-modified fast versus protein-formula-liquid diet. *Am. J. Clin. Nutr.* **1985**, *41*, 533–539. [CrossRef] [PubMed]
10. Fabricatore, A.N.; Wadden, T.A.; Higginbotham, A.J.; Faulconbridge, L.; Nguyen, A.M.; Heymsfield, S.B.; Faith, M.S. Intentional weight loss and changes in symptoms of depression: A systematic review and meta-analysis. *Int. J. Obes.* **2011**, *35*, 1363–1376. [CrossRef]
11. Sadeghirad, B.; Motaghipisheh, S.; Kolahdooz, F.; Zahedi, M.J.; Haghdoost, A. Islamic fasting and weight loss: A systematic review and meta-analysis. *Public Health Nutr.* **2014**, *17*, 396–406. [CrossRef] [PubMed]
12. Harris, L.; Hamilton, S.; Azevedo, L.B.; Olajide, J.; De Brún, C.; Waller, G.; Whittaker, V.; Sharp, T.; Lean, M.; Hankey, C.; et al. Intermittent fasting interventions for treatment of overweight and obesity in adults. *JBI Database Syst. Rev. Implement. Rep.* **2018**, *16*, 507–547. [CrossRef] [PubMed]
13. Guerrero, A.E.; Martín, I.S.M.; Vilar, E.G.; Martín, M.A.C. Effectiveness of an intermittent fasting diet versus continuous energy restriction on anthropometric measurements, body composition and lipid profile in overweight and obese adults: A meta-analysis. *Eur. J. Clin. Nutr.* **2021**, *75*, 1024–1039. [CrossRef] [PubMed]
14. De Cabo, R.; Mattson, M.P. Effects of intermittent fasting on health, aging, and disease. *N. Engl. J. Med.* **2019**, *381*, 2541–2551. [CrossRef] [PubMed]
15. Fond, G.; Macgregor, A.; Leboyer, M.; Michalsen, A. Fasting in mood disorders: Neurobiology and effectiveness. A review of the literature. *Psychiatry Res.* **2013**, *209*, 253–258. [CrossRef] [PubMed]
16. Gergelyfi, M.; Sanz-Arigita, E.J.; Solopchuk, O.; Dricot, L.; Jacob, B.; Zénon, A. Mental fatigue correlates with depression of task-related network and augmented DMN activity but spares the reward circuit. *NeuroImage* **2021**, *243*, 118532. [CrossRef]
17. Kahleova, H.; Belinova, L.; Hill, M.; Pelikanova, T. Do patients with type 2 diabetes still need to eat snacks? *Eur. J. Clin. Nutr.* **2015**, *69*, 755–756. [CrossRef]
18. NIH Study Quality Assessment Tools | NHLBI, NIH 2021. Available online: https://www.nhlbi.nih.gov/health-topics/study-quality-assessment-tools (accessed on 1 September 2021).
19. Nugraha, B.; Ghashang, S.K.; Hamdan, I.; Gutenbrunner, C. Effect of Ramadan fasting on fatigue, mood, sleepiness, and health-related quality of life of healthy young men in summer time in Germany: A prospective controlled study. *Appetite* **2017**, *111*, 38–45. [CrossRef]
20. Teng, N.I.M.F.; Shahar, S.; Manaf, Z.A.; Das, S.K.; Taha, C.S.C.; Ngah, W.Z.W. Efficacy of fasting calorie restriction on quality of life among aging men. *Physiol. Behav.* **2011**, *104*, 1059–1064. [CrossRef] [PubMed]
21. Hussin, N.M.; Shahar, S.; Teng, N.I.M.F.; Ngah, W.Z.W.; Das, S.K. Efficacy of Fasting and Calorie Restriction (FCR) on mood and depression among ageing men. *J. Nutr. Health Aging* **2013**, *17*, 674–680. [CrossRef] [PubMed]
22. Koushali, A.N.; Hajiamini, Z.; Ebadi, A.; Bayat, N.; Khamseh, F. Effect of Ramadan fasting on emotional reactions in nurses. *Iran. J. Nurs. Midwifery Res.* **2013**, *18*, 232–236.
23. Mousavi, S.A.; Rezaei, M.; Baghni, S.A.; Seifi, M. Effect of fasting on mental health in the general population of Kermanshah, Iran. *J. Nutr. Health* **2014**, *2*, 65–70.
24. Martin, C.K.; Bhapkar, M.; Pittas, A.G.; Pieper, C.F.; Das, S.K.; Williamson, D.A.; Scott, T.; Redman, L.M.; Stein, R.; Gilhooly, C.H.; et al. Effect of Calorie Restriction on Mood, Quality of Life, Sleep, and Sexual Function in Healthy Nonobese Adults. *JAMA Intern. Med.* **2016**, *176*, 743–752. [CrossRef] [PubMed]
25. Prehn, K.; Von Schwartzenberg, R.J.; Mai, K.; Zeitz, U.; Witte, A.V.; Hampel, D.; Szela, A.-M.; Fabian, S.; Grittner, U.; Spranger, J.; et al. Caloric Restriction in Older Adults—Differential Effects of Weight Loss and Reduced Weight on Brain Structure and Function. *Cereb. Cortex* **2016**, *27*, 1765–1778. [CrossRef] [PubMed]
26. Erdem, O. The investigation of the effects of Ramadan fasting on the mood state of healthy volunteer persons. *Fam. Pract. Palliat. CARE* **2018**, *3*, 1–6. [CrossRef]
27. Kessler, C.S.; Stange, R.; Schlenkermann, M.; Jeitler, M.; Michalsen, A.; Selle, A.; Raucci, F.; Steckhan, N. A nonrandomized controlled clinical pilot trial on 8 wk of intermittent fasting (24 h/wk). *Nutrition* **2018**, *46*, 143–152.e2. [CrossRef] [PubMed]
28. Al-Ozairi, E.; Alawadhi, M.M.; Al-Ozairi, A.; Taghadom, E.; Ismail, K.; Isamil, K. A prospective study of the effect of fasting during the month of Ramadan on depression and diabetes distress in people with type 2 diabetes. *Diabetes Res. Clin. pract.* **2019**, *153*, 145–149. [CrossRef] [PubMed]

29. Secades-Villa, R.; González-Roz, A.; García-Pérez, Á.; Becoña, E. Psychological, pharmacological, and combined smoking cessation interventions for smokers with current depression: A systematic review and meta-analysis. *PLoS ONE* **2017**, *12*, e0188849. [CrossRef]
30. Ioannou, M.; Wartenberg, C.; Greenbrook, J.T.V.; Larson, T.; Magnusson, K.; Schmitz, L.; Sjögren, P.; Stadig, I.; Szabó, Z.; Steingrimsson, S. Sleep deprivation as treatment for depression: Systematic review and meta-analysis. *Acta Psychiatr. Scand.* **2021**, *143*, 22–35. [CrossRef]
31. Silva, D.A.; Coutinho, E.D.S.F.; Ferriani, L.O.; Viana, M.C. Depression subtypes and obesity in adults: A systematic review and meta-analysis. *Obes. Rev.* **2019**, *21*, e12966. [CrossRef] [PubMed]
32. Grigolon, R.B.; Trevizol, A.P.; Gerchman, F.; Bambokian, A.D.; Magee, T.; McIntyre, R.S.; Gomes, F.A.; Brietzke, E.; Mansur, R.B. Is Obesity A Determinant Of Success With Pharmacological Treatment For Depression? A Systematic Review, Meta-Analysis And Meta-Regression. *J. Affect. Disord.* **2021**, *287*, 54–68. [CrossRef] [PubMed]
33. Garcia, G.D.; Pompeo, D.A.; Eid, L.P.; Cesarino, C.B.; Pinto, M.H.; Gonçalves, L.W.P. Relationship between anxiety, depressive symptoms and compulsive overeating disorder in patients with cardiovascular diseases. *Rev. Lat.-Am. Enferm.* **2018**, *26*, 3040. [CrossRef] [PubMed]
34. Ensminger, D.C.; Salvador-Pascual, A.; Arango, B.G.; Allen, K.N.; Vázquez-Medina, J.P. Fasting ameliorates oxidative stress: A review of physiological strategies across life history events in wild vertebrates. *Comp. Biochem. Physiol. Part A Mol. Integr. Physiol.* **2021**, *256*, 110929. [CrossRef] [PubMed]

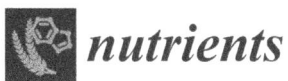

Article

Dietary Patterns, Eating Behavior, and Nutrient Intakes of Spanish Preschool Children with Autism Spectrum Disorders

Julio Plaza-Diaz [1,2,3,†], Katherine Flores-Rojas [4,5,†], María José de la Torre-Aguilar [4,*], Antonio Rafael Gomez-Fernández [4], Pilar Martín-Borreguero [6], Juan Luis Perez-Navero [4,7], Angel Gil [1,5,8] and Mercedes Gil-Campos [4,5]

1. Department of Biochemistry and Molecular Biology II, School of Pharmacy, University of Granada, 18071 Granada, Spain; jrplaza@ugr.es (J.P.-D.); agil@ugr.es (A.G.)
2. Instituto de Investigación Biosanitaria IBS.GRANADA, Complejo Hospitalario Universitario de Granada, 18014 Granada, Spain
3. Children's Hospital of Eastern Ontario Research Institute, Ottawa, ON K1H 8L1, Canada
4. Pediatric Research and Metabolism Unit, Maimónides Institute for Biomedical Research of Córdoba (IMIBIC), Reina Sofia University Hospital, University of Córdoba, Av. Menéndez Pidal, s/n, 14010 Córdoba, Spain; katherine1.flores@gmail.com (K.F.-R.); antoniogofedez@hotmail.com (A.R.G.-F.); juanpereznavero@hotmail.com (J.L.P.-N.); mercedes_gil_campos@yahoo.es (M.G.-C.)
5. CIBEROBN (Physiopathology of Obesity and Nutrition), Instituto de Salud Carlos III (ISCIII), 28029 Madrid, Spain
6. Department of Child and Adolescent Clinical Psychiatry and Psychology, Maimónides Institute for Biomedical Research of Córdoba (IMIBIC), Reina Sofia University Hospital, Av. Menéndez Pidal, s/n, 14010 Córdoba, Spain; pmartin.psicologa@gmail.com
7. Centre for Biomedical Research on Rare Diseases (CIBERER), ISCIII, 28029 Madrid, Spain
8. Biomedical Research Center, Institute of Nutrition and Food Technology "José Mataix", University of Granada, Parque Tecnológico de la Salud, Avenida del Conocimiento, s/n, 18016 Granada, Spain
* Correspondence: delatorremj4@gmail.com; Tel.: +34-957736467
† These authors contributed equally to this work.

Abstract: Eating behavior problems are characteristic of children with autism spectrum disorders (ASD) with a highly restricted range of food choices, which may pose an associated risk of nutritional problems. Hence, detailed knowledge of the dietary patterns (DPs) and nutrient intakes of ASD patients is necessary to carry out intervention strategies if required. The present study aimed to determine the DPs and macro-and micronutrient intakes in a sample of Spanish preschool children with ASD compared to typically developing control children. Fifty-four children with ASD (two to six years of age) diagnosed with ASD according to the Diagnostic Manual-5 criteria), and a control group of 57 typically developing children of similar ages were recruited. A validated food frequency questionnaire was used, and the intake of energy and nutrients was estimated through three non-consecutive 24-h dietary registrations. DPs were assessed using principal component analysis and hierarchical clustering analysis. Children with ASD exhibited a DP characterized by high energy and fat intakes and a low intake of vegetables and fruits. Likewise, meat intake of any type, both lean and fatty, was associated with higher consumption of fish and dietary fat. Furthermore, the increased consumption of dairy products was associated with increased consumption of cereals and pasta. In addition, they had frequent consumption of manufactured products with poor nutritional quality, e.g., beverages, sweets, snacks and bakery products. The percentages of children with ASD complying with the adequacy of nutrient intakes were higher for energy, saturated fat, calcium, and vitamin C, and lower for iron, iodine, and vitamins of group B when compared with control children. In conclusion, this study emphasizes the need to assess the DPs and nutrient intakes of children with ASD to correct their alterations and discard some potential nutritional diseases.

Keywords: autism spectrum disorders; disabled children; food and nutrition; feeding behavior

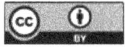

1. Introduction

Autism Spectrum Disorders (ASD) are neurodevelopmental disorders characterized by disturbances in communication and social interaction and by the presence of restricted, repetitive patterns of behaviors, activities, and interests. These alterations are present from early childhood, although some difficulties may not manifest until the environment's demands exceed the child's capacity [1]. Most studies coincide with a significant increase in the prevalence of ASD, which does not seem to be explained by improving the detection systems. For 2016, ASD prevalence in the USA was 18.5 per 1000 (one in 54) children aged eight years, and ASD was 4.3 times as prevalent among boys as among girls [2]. It must therefore be considered a serious public health problem.

Children with ASD frequently have significant eating difficulties with a highly restricted range of food choices [3], and there is consensus that children with ASD have selective dietary patterns (DPs), food neophobia and sensory issues [4]. Indeed, the Diagnostic Manual-5 (DSM-5) now includes sensory symptoms in the diagnostic criteria for ASD, such as food selectivity [1]. Eating behavior problems are characteristics of ASD [5–7]. The dietary complications are more common among children with ASD than among the population during the first year of life from the time of introducing the complementary foods [8]. The rejection of solid foods is very frequent, and the introduction of foods with new textures, consistencies, and flavors tends to be difficult, so they preferentially consume the same foods in a repetitive manner [9,10]. Those behaviours do not seem to influence their growth long-term [4]. Still, they generate a great deal of family anxiety, becoming one of the main concerns of caregivers and family members [11,12]. Although these behaviours usually improve with time [13], the possible nutritional repercussions and the important social limitations are relevant and sensory goals should be included in treatment objectives for children with ASD [11].

The origin of eating behavior alterations is not entirely clear. Among some of the theories that can explain this phenomenon, the following stand out: (1) cognitive/behavioral alterations [14–16]; (2) sensory alterations [4,16,17]; and (3) gastrointestinal disturbances [18,19]. Eating problems in children and adolescents with ASD represent a concern for parents and caregivers and a potential cause of health issues. However, studies are diverse, presenting differences in the methodological steps, so their outcomes are hard to compare [20]. Some investigations have reviewed the consumption of children with ASD compared to those with typical development and determined some nutritional preferences of children with ASD. In general, they found stronger preferences for energy-dense foods like snacks, sweets, sugary beverages and juice in children with ASD. In contrast, children with ASD tend to eat less from food groups like vegetables, fruit and dairy products than children with typical development [21].

Without curative treatments and with these eating behavior alterations [22], the use of nutritional supplements and alternative medicine, which is widely used among families of ASD patients, has been greatly encouraged [23,24] when seeking clinical improvement. However, the use of nutritional supplements e.g., those containing omega-3 fatty acids [25], multivitamins, as well as a gluten-free casein-free diet [26], is not supported by the current scientific evidence, and it should not be generally recommended.

It has been suggested that the identification and development of nutritional assessment indicators that serve as early warning signs during routine practice are of interest [4]. Indeed, the present study aimed to determine the feeding behavior, DPs, and macro-and micronutrient intakes in a sample of Spanish preschool children with ASD compared to typically developing control children of the same age.

2. Material and Methods

2.1. Study Design and Subjects

The present work is part of an observational and case-control study described elsewhere [27]. ASD patients from two to six years old in a specialized Unit for ASD in a third level hospital (Reina Sofia University Hospital, Cordoba, Spain) and diagnosed according to DSM-5 criteria and validated by the Autism Diagnostic Observation Schedule (ADOS) score were recruited. A group of healthy children of similar age to that of the ASD group that came to the hospital for minimal surgery interventions with a normal detailed clinical history, general examination, anthropometric assessment, and control analysis to rule out any pathology was used as a control group. Both groups lived in the same urban area of Córdoba (Spain), with families in similar economic and sociocultural situations and close environmental exposure. Exclusion criteria were receiving medication for ASD comorbidities and any other pathology, be receiving or have received any nutritional supplement in the last 12 months; undertaking specific diets for therapeutic purposes in the previous 12 months e.g., celiac disease; and having a percentile higher than p97 or lower than p3 in the recommended tables of anthropometry of the Spanish child population [28,29].

The diagnosis of ASD was assessed following the clinical criteria of the DSM-5 and confirmed with the completion of the ADOS. An initial sample of 55 children with ASD (46 males and 9 females) between two and six years of age was recruited, following the inclusion criteria. During the recruitment phase, a male was excluded because he was diagnosed with celiac disease (n = 54). Fifty-seven healthy children, after normal results as noted above, were also included in the study as a control group.

The present study was approved by the Clinical Research and Bioethics Committee of the Hospital Reina Sofía, Cordoba, Spain. It was conducted in full compliance with the fundamental principles established in the Declaration of Helsinki. The data relating to the ASD patients were collected at the time they were recruited into the study. The recruited subjects were incorporated into the study after all the criteria for inclusion were fulfilled, and informed written consent was obtained from the children's legal guardians.

2.2. Variables and Data Collection

In the recruited patients diagnosed with ASD and in the control subjects, a detailed history and general physical examination was performed.

A previously modified, adapted and validated food frequency questionnaire (FFQ) with the portion sizes and food groups usually consumed by the Spanish child population was used [30]. The adequacy of food consumption was evaluated using the Nutritional Objectives of the Consensus Document of the Spanish Community Nutrition Society; these questionnaires included one item about the dietary type and amount of supplementation [31].

The intake of energy and nutrients was estimated from the data obtained through three non-consecutive 24-h dietary registrations (24-h-DR), registered by parents, including two weekdays and one weekend day, following the Guidance on the EU Menu Methodology of the European Food Safety Agency (EFSA) [32]. Mean daily intakes of energy and nutrients were calculated by using the computer software of the Center of Endocrinology and Clinical Research, University of Valladolid, Institute of Studies on Health Sciences of Castilla and Leon, Spain (IENVA) (https://calcdieta.ienva.org/, accessed on 1 September 2021).

2.3. Statistical Analysis

2.3.1. General Analyses

The sample size for the study was calculated assuming a 30% difference in the mean for one of the main study variables (plasma level of docosahexaenoic acid) between children with ASD and healthy children, an α error = 0.05, a power of 0.90 (β error of 0.1) and 5% of dropout during the follow-up of the study. For these calculations, data from recent studies were used, considering that the percentages expected would be similar to several studies carried out in populations with similar characteristics to those of children with ASD. Data were expressed as mean ± standard deviation or median plus interquartile range, depending on whether each variable's values followed a normal distribution or not. The Shapiro-Wilk normality test was used to determine the normality of variables. The comparison between the groups was carried out using the Student's *t*-test for continuous variables when the distributions were normal and the Mann-Whitney U test when the distributions did not follow the normality. The differences between the frequencies of the sexes were studied by means of the Chi-square test. For the statistical analysis of the data, the computer program IBM SPSS 25.0 (IBM Corp., Armonk, NY, USA) was used.

2.3.2. Dietary Patterns

A principal component analysis (PCA) was accomplished to identify underlying DPs using each individual's serving average from nine food groups as input variables [31]. These food groups considered in this study were as follows: "milk and dairy products (e.g., milk, yogurt, cheese, and milkshakes)", "cereals and pasta (e.g., bread, cereal bars, and rice)", "fatty meat and derivates", "fats", "snacks, sweets, bakery and pastry (e.g., chocolate, cookies, ice cream, candies, and bakery products)", "fruits and vegetables", "beverages", "fish and shellfish (e.g., white fish, bluefish, and shellfish)", and "lean meat and eggs". This mathematical model calculates new variables (principal components) that account for the variability in the food group's data and enables the study of covariances or correlations between variables. We interpreted only components with eigenvalues over one and factor loadings with an absolute value higher than 0.4 (which explains around 16% of variance) as the significance of factor loading depends on the sample size. A high factor score for a given pattern indicated a high consumption of the foods constituting that food factor, and a low score indicated a low intake of those foods.

The Kaiser–Meyer–Olkin (KMO) and Bartlett test of sphericity were applied to assess the sampling adequacy. KMO values >0.50 were considered. Communalities were estimated using the squared multiple correlations of each variable with all others. We retained variables with communalities higher than 0.5. Factors were orthogonally rotated (the Varimax option) to maximize the dispersion of loading within factors, facilitating interpretability. Radar maps were used to display data in the form of a two-dimensional map of nine food groups represented on axes starting from the same point.

2.3.3. Dietary Patterns with Clustering Analysis

A two-step cluster analysis procedure was conducted for the automatic selection of the best number of clusters that would otherwise not be apparent on the FFQ variables. Three clusters were assumed to be the optimum number. Later, unsupervised hierarchical clustering analysis was applied to construct clusters of subjects with similar characteristics using the "pheatmap" R software package. The distance matrix was defined by Euclidean distances, and Ward's method was used as linkage criteria to group the clusters. The agglomerative coefficient, calculated by the Agnes function, was always higher than 0.85.

Heat maps were used to visualize hierarchical clustering, which allowed us to simultaneously picture clusters of subjects and features. Hierarchical clustering was done of both the rows and the columns of the data matrix, which were re-ordered according to the hierarchical clustering result, putting similar observations close to each other. The blocks of 'high' and 'low' values are adjacent in the data matrix. A red-blue color scheme was applied for the visualization to help to find the variables that appear to be characteristic for each subject cluster.

3. Results

3.1. Subjects Characteristics

Table 1 shows the control group's demographic characteristics, comprising 57 healthy children and the ASD group, including 54 patients. The proportion of boys with ASD was higher than that of girls. There were no significant differences in weight, height, and body mass index (BMI) between the two groups.

Table 1. Demographic and anthropometric characteristics of the group of children with autism spectrum disorders and the control healthy group.

Variables	Control (n = 57)	ASD (n = 54)	p-Value
Age (months)	51.5 (33–60)	42 (33–51)	0.07
Sex (male)	43 (75%)	45 (83.33%)	0.28
Weight (kg)	17.3 ± 2.5	16.7 ± 3.5	0.3
Height (cm)	106.3 ± 8.3	103.4 ± 9.7	0.6
BMI (kg/m^2)	16.1 ± 1.7	15.9 ± 1.9	0.4

ASD: Autism Spectrum Disorders; BMI: Body Mass Index. The data have been expressed as mean ± standard deviation and absolute frequencies (%).

3.2. Food Group Consumption According to Food Frequency Questionnaires and Adequacy to the Spanish Society of Community Nutrition (SENC) Dietary Guidelines

Children with ASD consumed more cereals and pasta, and milk and dairy products than the control group; in contrast, ASD children consumed fewer lean meat, eggs, and beverages. The questionnaires highlighted the consumption, in shredded form, preferably of chicken or beef with vegetables, and to a lesser extent fatty meats and fish (Table 2).

Table 2. Food group consumption according to food frequency questionnaires in Spanish preschool children with autism spectrum disorders (ASD).

Food Groups	Control (n = 57)	ASD (n = 54)
Cereals and pasta (s/d)	2.6 ± 1.0	4.6 ± 1.5 *
Fruits and vegetables (s/d)	2.0 ± 1.2	2.2 ± 0.9
Milk and dairy products (s/d)	3.2 ± 1.3	4.3 ± 1.6 *
Fish and shellfish (s/wk)	2.6 ± 1.1	2.5 ± 1.2
Lean meat and eggs (s/wk)	4.6 ± 1.4	2.0 ± 0.5 *
Fatty meats and derivatives (s/wk)	3.6 ± 2.3	2.8 ± 1.5
Fats (s/d)	2.8 ± 1.8	2.3 ± 0.6
Beverages (s/wk)	6.2 ± 3.1	4.1 ± 1.0 *
Snacks, sweets, bakery and pastry (s/wk)	5.5 ± 3.2	4.6 ± 2.8

Food servings are shown in mean ± standard deviation in servings per day (s/d) or servings per week (s/wk). Statistical differences were calculated using the U-Mann Whitney test between ASD and the control groups (* $p < 0.05$).

Table 3 shows the food group consumption according to food frequency questionnaires and adherence to the Spanish Society of Community Nutrition (SENC) dietary guidelines for preschool children with ASD compared with the control group. A higher percentage of ASD children consumed four to six servings per day of cereals and pasta compared with the control group. A significantly higher percentage of ASD children consumed more than six servings of milk and dairy products compared with the control children. A high percentage of ASD children consumed less than three servings/wk of lean meats and eggs compared to the control children.

In contrast, both groups of children consumed an excess of fatty meats and their foodstuffs. The majority of ASD children consumed 2–3 servings of fat daily, whereas 22.8% of the control children consumed more than 3 servings/d. Finally, more than 85% of both ASD and control children consumed more servings than those recommended for beverages, snacks, sweets, bakery, and pastry.

Table 3. Percentage of food group consumption (in servings per day or week) according to food frequency questionnaires and adequacy to the Spanish Society of Community Nutrition (SENC) dietary guidelines of preschool children with ASD compared with a healthy control group.

Food Groups (SENC Guidelines)	Control (n = 57)			ASD (n = 54)			p-Value
Cereals and pasta (4–6 s/d)	<4 82.5	4–6 17.5	>6 0	<4 25.9	4–6 63	>6 11.1	<0.001
Fruits and vegetables (≥5 s/d)	<3 87.7		>3 12.3	<3 96.3		>3 3.7	0.098
Milk and dairy products (2–4 s/d)	<2 10.5	2–4 71.9	>4 17.5	<2 3.7	2–4 59.3	>4 37	0.041
Fish and shellfish (3–4 s/wk)	>3 49.1	3–4 45.6	>4 5.3	>3 63	3–4 29.6	>4 7.4	0.22
Lean meat and eggs (3–5 s/wk)	<3 7.0	3–5 61.4	>5 31.6	<3 94.4	3–5 5.6	>5 0	<0.001
Fatty meats and derivatives (≤1 s/wk)	0 1.8	1 10.5	>2 87.7	0 1.9	1 16.7	>2 81.5	0.637
Fats (2–3 s/d) *	<2 15.8	2–3 61.4	>3 22.8	<2 3.7	2–3 94.4	>3 1.9	<0.001
Beverages (≤1 s/wk)	0 0	1 1.8	>2 98.2	0 0	1 0	>2 100	0.328
Snacks, sweets, bakery and pastry (≤1 s/wk)	0 7	1 3.5	>2 89.5	0 3.7	1 7.4	>2 88.9	0.511

SENC recommended food servings are shown in servings per day (s/d) or servings per week (s/wk), and the frequency of food consumption data are expressed as percentages (below). Statistical differences were calculated using a Chi-square test * Includes mostly olive oil for meal preparation.

3.3. Dietary Patterns

Figure 1 depicts the DPs of ASD and control children evaluated through PCA's bi-dimensional plots related to the major food groups consumed. The two dimensions, Dim1 (X-axis) and Dim2 (Y-axis) explained 22.5% and 17.5% of the total variance, respectively. Most ASD subjects separated well from the control subjects because of the increased consumption of cereals and pasta and milk and dairy products and the relatively lower consumption of lean meat and egg, fatty meats and derivatives, fish and shellfish, beverages, snacks, sweets, and bakery and pastry, compared with the control children.

A three-dimensional PCA was used to maximize the diet's predominant food groups' information. The combination of food group variables with the greatest amount of variability is the first principal component. The following components (second and third principal components) describe the maximum amount of remaining variability.

Figure 2 shows the DPs extracted from the three-dimensional PCA of nine major food groups for the control group (Panel A) and children with ASD (Panel B). In the control children, the first component was associated with a healthy pattern that included fruit and vegetables, fish, and lean meats and eggs. The second component was related to the consumption of milk and dairy, cereals and pasta to snacks, sweets, bakery, and pastry and beverages. The third component associated a high consumption of fat with low consumption of fatty meats and their derivatives. In contrast, the ASD group's first component showed an unhealthy pattern characterized by a high relationship between low consumption of fruits and vegetables and increased consumption of snacks, sweets, bakery, and pastry, and beverages. The second component was described by the associated consumption of different meats, fish, and fat types. The third component included the related consumption of milk and dairy products and cereals and pasta.

Clusters of subjects classified based on their dietary characteristics are shown in a heat-map (Figure 3). There were two main clusters of children (columns) and three main dietary variables (rows) identified by the clustering algorithm. All ASD children, excepting one subject, and all healthy children, were classified into two distinct clusters (blue for the ASD and red for the control population in Figure 3. Within the first food cluster, ASD children exhibited low consumption of lean meat and eggs, snacks, sweets, bakery, and pastry, fats, and beverages compared with the control population's children. In contrast, ASD children showed higher milk and dairy consumption and cereals and pasta for the second food cluster. In the third food cluster, the consumption of fatty meats and their derivatives, fruits and vegetables, and fish varied for different subjects in the ASD and control children.

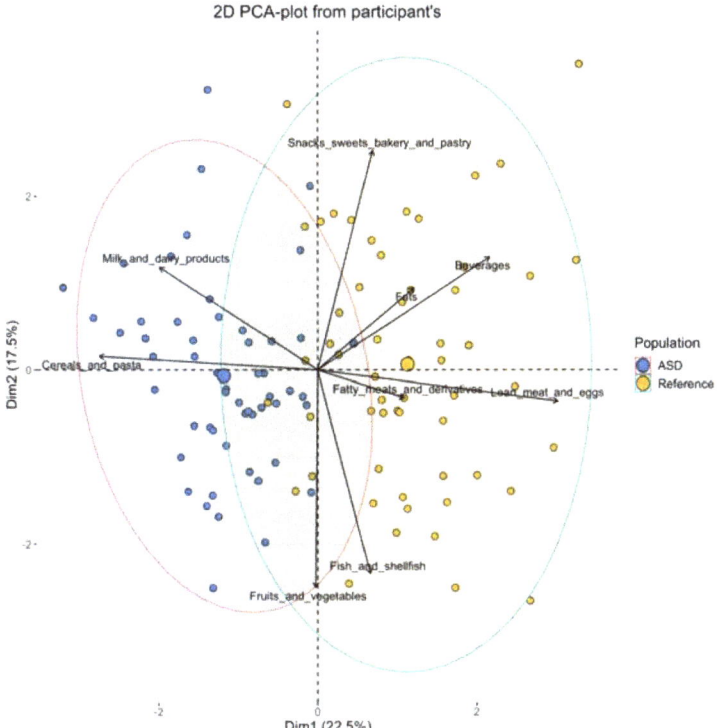

Figure 1. Principal component analysis (PCA) plot in the control and the children with autism spectrum disorders (ASD) according to the intake of major food groups determined by a standardized food frequency questionnaire.

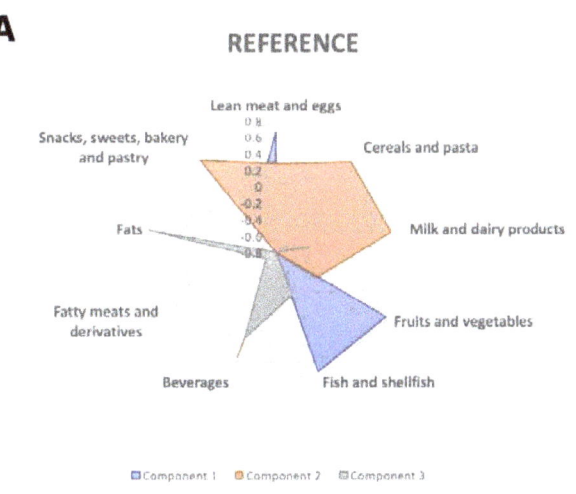

Figure 2. *Cont.*

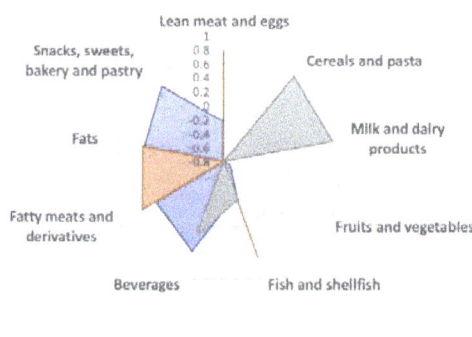

Figure 2. Dietary patterns extracted from the three-dimension principal component analysis of 9 major food groups. (**A**) Control group ($n = 57$), (**B**) Children with ASD ($n = 54$).

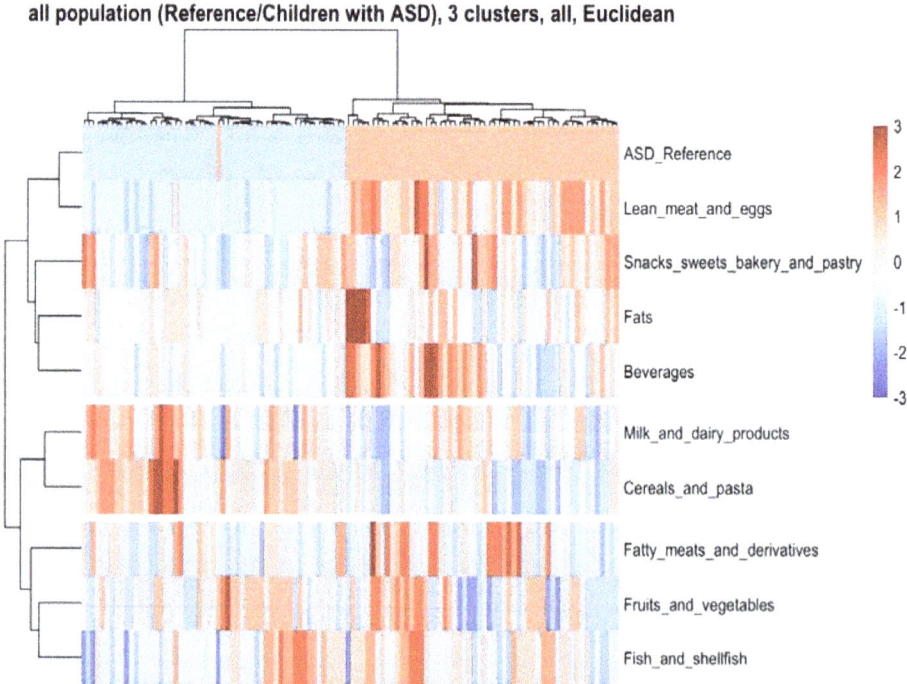

Figure 3. Clusters of subjects and dietary and lifestyle variables were identified via hierarchical clustering in control and ASD groups. The clusters are visually separated by longitudinal marks on vertical and horizontal faces (clusters of subjects and dietary variables, respectively). The vertical and horizontal dendrograms denote the relationship between the clusters, i.e., similar observations. The color bar refers to levels above (red) or below (blue) the mean intake of the dietary variable or means scores of food groups. Increased color intensities indicate larger differences around the mean. For the ASD control variable, ASD children are represented by the color blue and children of the control group by the color red.

3.4. Eating Behavior

Of the ASD 54 patients, 42% tolerated solid foods, whereas 58% tolerated only pureed foods. When comparing the number of servings for the different food groups within the ASD patient groups (solid vs. pureed), significant differences were obtained in vegetables, fruit, fish, and fatty meats ($p < 0.05$) (Figure 4). All control children tolerated solid foods.

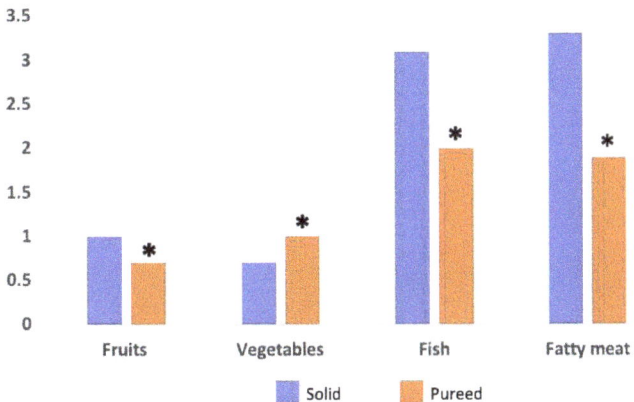

Figure 4. The average consumption of solids and pureed foods in Spanish preschool children with autism spectrum disorders for selected food groups (vegetables and fruit are expressed in servings/day, and fish and meat in servings/week). * $p < 0.05$.

3.5. Adequacy of Nutrient Intakes to the European Food Safety Authority (EFSA) Recommendations

To assess nutrient adequacy, individual usual intake was compared to the current recommendations of adequate intake (AI) and reference intake range (RI) defined by EFSA [30]. Table 4 shows the percentages of children meeting and not meeting the EFSA recommendations for energy, macronutrients, minerals, and vitamins.

The majority of ASD children had an adequate energy intake, while about 23% of the control group did not reach the EFSA recommendations. Both ASD and the control group had a higher intake of protein than recommended by EFSA. The intake of carbohydrates was similar in the two groups of children, with more than 70% following the recommendations. Nevertheless, the intake of sugars in both groups was higher than recommended in the majority of children. In contrast, the recommended intake of fiber was not reached by about 51% of ASD children compared with only 23.4% in the healthy control group, although only a statistical trend was found ($p = 0.085$). Besides, the percentage of ASD children who had an intake of saturated fat above the guidelines was higher compared with that of the control children. The intake of total polyunsaturated fatty acids was similar in both groups of children. Even the intakes of essential fatty acids [linoleic acid (LA) and α-linolenic acid (LNA)] were similar; the average energy intake was lower than that recommended by the EFSA (LA: 1.25% and 1.13%; LNA 0.13% and 0.13%, respectively). The average intake of EPA + DHA was about 0.3 g/d for the control and 0.15 g/d for ASD children, which is close to the EFSA guidelines.

About 79% of ASD children had an adequate calcium intake compared with only about 50% in the control group. Adequacies of phosphorus, magnesium, and potassium intake were similar in both groups. However, most of the subjects in both groups did not reach the AI for magnesium. Similarly, the iron, zinc, copper, and manganese intakes were lower than the corresponding AI in most ASD and in the control group. The adequacy of intake was lower in ASD children than in the control group; in fact, 100.0% of ASD children did not meet the AI for iodine (Table 4).

Table 4. Adequacy of nutrient intake to the European Food Safe Authority (EFSA) recommendations of Spanish preschool children with autism spectrum disorders (ASD) compared with a healthy control group.

Variables	Control Group (n = 57)			Children ASD (n = 47)			p-Value
	Percentage below AI or RI	Percentage within RI	Percentage over AI or RI	Percentage below AI or RI	Percentage within RI	Percentage over AI or RI	
Energy	22.8		77.2	2.1		97.9	0.002
Proteins	0		100	0		100	1
Carbohydrates	14.3	76.8	8.9	21.3	76.6	2.1	0.254
Sugars	15.8		84.2	6.4		93.6	0.135
Fiber	50.9		49.1	34.0		66.6	0.085
Fats	50.9	28.1	21.1	23.4	38.3	38.3	0.014
Polyunsaturated fats	68.4		31.6	72.3		27.7	0.664
Saturated fats	47.4		52.6	23.4		76.6	0.012
Potassium	31.6		68.4	34.0		66.6	0.79
Calcium	49.1		50.1	21.3		78.7	0.003
Phosphorus	14.0		86	19.1		80.9	0.483
Magnesium	98.2		1.8	100		0	0.362
Iron	80.7		19.3	97.9		2.1	0.006
Zinc	70.2		29.8	80.9		19.1	0.211
Copper	96.5		3.5	100		0	0.195
Selenium	15.8		84.2	29.8		70.2	0.087
Manganese	100		0	100		0	1
Iodine	63.2		36.8	100		0	<0.001
Vitamin A	61.4		38.6	57.4		42.6	0.682
Vitamin D	91.2		8.8	95.7		4.3	0.36
Vitamin E	94.7		5.3	85.1		14.9	0.097
Vitamin K	57.9		42.1	44.7		55.3	0.179
Vitamin B1	56.1		43.9	91.5		8.5	<0.001
Vitamin B2	24.6		75.4	68.1		31.9	<0.001
Vitamin B3	96.5		3.5	100		0	0.195
Vitamin B6	33.3		66.7	53.2		46.8	0.041
Vitamin B9	91.2		8.8	91.5		8.5	0.962
Vitamin B12	24.6		75.4	48.9		51.1	0.01
Vitamin C	42.1		57.9	21.3		78.7	0.024

Nutrient adequacy was assessed by comparison of estimated usual individual intakes with the recommendations of adequate intake (AI) and reference intake range (RI) defined by EFSA [30]. Data are expressed as percentages of children below, within and over the recommended EFSA intake range for each nutrient. Percentage differences between ASD and control children were calculated using the Chi-square test.

Regarding the vitamins, the usual individual intakes of vitamins D, E and B9 were below the recommended AI in most of ASD and control children. The intakes of vitamin A and K were similar in both groups, with about one half following the recommendations. Finally, we observed significantly higher percentages of ASD children that did not meet the EFSA guidelines for vitamin B1, B2, B6, and B12 when compared with the control children.

4. Discussion

The major findings of the present study were: (1) children with ASD showed a DP characterized by relatively high consumption of cereals, pasta and dairy products, and a small intake of lean meat and eggs compared with the SENC guidelines [31]; (2) all children (control and ASD) consumed little fruit, vegetables, and fish. Instead, they ingested high amounts of fatty meat and its derivatives, as well as drinks, snacks, sweets, and baked goods confectionery. In particular, in children with ASD, the high intake of snacks, sweets, and bakery was associated with increased consumption of beverages and fat and lower consumption of fruits and vegetables; (3) the intake of meat of any type, both lean and fatty, was associated with higher consumption of fish and dietary fat. Also, the increased consumption of dairy products was associated with high consumption of cereals and pasta; (4) ASD children were grouped in a well-differentiated cluster from that of their control peers; (5) only about one-half of the children with ASD tolerated solid foods; (6) compared with control children, the percentages of ASD children complying with the adequacy of nutrient intakes were higher for energy, fat, saturated fat, calcium and vitamin C, and lower for fiber, iron, iodine, and vitamins of group B.

Families have related excessive consumption of cereals and dairy to an increased worsening of symptoms of ASD. However, systematic reviews on the gluten- and casein-free diet (GCFD) indicate that the evidence is insufficient to support or refute it [33–36]. Therefore, today GCFD for children with ASD cannot be recommended unless they are appropriately diagnosed with an allergy or intolerance to a certain compound or allergen. Instead, improvement of the DPs should be promoted by increasing consumption of fruits and vegetables, lean meat and fish, and decreasing consumption of enriched sugar and fatty food products, avoiding restricted diets unless there is a medical indication after a clear diagnosis of allergy or intolerance. In our study, even though having carried out a restriction diet for the treatment of ASD in the last 12 months was considered an exclusion criterion, none of the families interviewed reported using such diets.

Common DPs in children with ASD include a strong preference for processed foods, snacks, and starches coinciding with a bias against fruits and vegetables [37–39].

Some studies have shown that a DP with a low content of fibers (from legumes, nuts, and others) is associated with a reduced feeling of satiety during meals [40]. In addition, a higher intake of high energy density food, such as sweet cereals, sweets, and sugary drinks, constitutes an eating DP of high energy intake in all children. However, it is significant to note that this high-risk DP is more prominent among children with ASD, since their specificities in the consumption of some food groups lead them to a DP that diverges even further from the dietary guidelines (e.g., SENC guidelines) [21]. In the present work, except for dairy products, a relatively high proportion of children with ASD complied with the recommended food consumption guidelines of the SENC for pediatrics. In terms of food intake in ASD patients, there are some difficulties to consider which are not only related to their low tolerance of solid food but also with regard to their cognitive or behavioral rigidity, which determines a tendency in these patients to remain in a stable environment, and therefore makes the introduction of new foods difficult [16]. They also have difficulty in accepting certain textures, with alterations in palatability and also problems chewing and swallowing [41]. The intake of fruits and vegetables was lower than that recommended, mimicking what is usual in the whole Spanish population [42–45]. In agreement with our results, a study involving a sample of 70 children with ASD with severe food selectivity, i.e., complete omission of one or more food groups (e.g., fruit, vegetable, protein, grain, dairy) or consuming a narrow range of items weekly (e.g., five or fewer total food items) found that 67% of the sample omitted vegetables and 27% omitted fruits [46].

One aspect of interest is the higher consumption of snacks, sweets, and baked goods in ASD patients compared with the SENC recommendations. However, the families reported that snacks were used as a positive reinforcement in psychoeducational therapies that these patients usually carry out. Besides that, these foods are sometimes used to introduce patients to solid foods in those with low tolerance. Even though the ingestion of snacks is not recommended except occasionally, we are aware of the importance of psychoeducational treatments based on selectivity towards some foods, including snacks [47]. Hence, although a flexible attitude about the ingestion of this type of food in ASD children is understandable, the high consumption of snacks, sweets, and baked goods in all Spanish children has been repeatedly reported [42–45], and should be modified.

Other authors have also reported alterations in eating behavior patterns in ASD. Compared to children with typical development, preschoolers with ASD consumed fewer vegetables, fish, and eggs, while primary school children consumed fewer legumes, cheese/yogurt, olive oil, citrus fruits, and more meat [21]. In terms of food tolerance, more than half of our children with ASD consumed a high percentage of pureed foods, particularly fruits, vegetables, fish, and fatty meats, despite being over two years old, which is when the bulk of the foods and modes of consumption of an adult have already been incorporated [48]. Indeed, the families mentioned they usually had jars of comminuted food, preferably chicken or beef with vegetables, and to a lesser extent fatty meats and fish.

A recent study demonstrates that food selectivity and mealtime problems are common issues in preschoolers, school-age children, and adolescents with ASD, and they are associated with a higher frequency of gastrointestinal (GI) symptoms [49,50]. In our sample, at least in part, the increased consumption of shredded foods as well as the use of soft foods, e.g., porridges made by cereals with milk, and homogenized foods, might be due to the presence of minor GI symptoms.

Regarding nutrient intake, results in different studies are affected by many environmental and cultural factors. Sharp et al. (2013) [15] and Esteban-Figuerola et al. (2019) [51] have reported a lower intake of calcium and protein in autistic children compared with a control group, while here the intake of protein was higher than the recommendations and similar to the general population [15,51]. Likewise, the intake of fat for a majority of the ASD children complied with the recommendations, and even the intake of saturated fat was higher than in their control peers.

Essential fatty acids, LA and LNA, and their long-chain PUFA derivatives, mainly arachidonic acid (AA) and docosahexaenoic acid (DHA), play essential roles in growth and neurodevelopment, as well as in the prevention of diseases. Furthermore, low DHA levels have been associated with impaired language and motor skills in infants and children [52]. It has been suggested that children with ASD may be deficient in n-3 PUFA; in that sense, some studies have shown altered phospholipid–fatty acid compositions in plasma and red blood cells from children with ASD [53,54] and that dietary supplementation with EPA and DHA may contribute to improving the symptomatology [55–59]. However, the available data in this regard are scarce and often contradictory [34,59–62]. In contrast to other studies, in our sample the average daily intake of EPA + DHA in ASD children was about 0.125 g/d, close to the recommendations of the EFSA and other international entities e.g., FAO-OMS [63], and that value did not differ significantly from that observed in the control children. So these data do not seem to justify the use of omega 3 as a treatment in ASD, at least in Spain, where the familiar consumption of fish is traditionally higher compared to other countries [64]. In cases with low intake of fish, it could be recommended to plan a therapeutic test with supplementations to analyze blood levels fatty acids beforehand

Several studies have shown that children with ASD have inadequate micronutrient intakes [65,66], and they are at particular risk for specific inadequacies of vitamins and minerals such as calcium, magnesium, vitamin D, and vitamin E [39,46,51]. Children with ASD have also demonstrated low levels of folate, vitamins B6, and B12, which have been associated with simultaneous B6, B9, and B12 deficiencies leading to the accumulation of homocysteine [59,67]. In relation to the intake of calcium, our study shows different results compared with that of the Esteban-Figuerola et al. meta analysis (2019) [51]. In the present study, patients with ASD had a higher calcium intake than typically developing controls. This difference seems to be due to the increased consumption of dairy products reported by most of the families. This result can be contrasted with the tendency to use restriction diets in these patients, mainly GFCD, as described earlier, which implies the withdrawal of milk from the diet [33]. On the other hand, the limited intake of some micronutrients involved in the metabolism of 1-carbon fragments, such as folate, vitamin B12, and vitamin B6, may be critical because they contribute to the processes of DNA and histone methylation, which in turn influence the expression of numerous genes involved in neurodevelopment [68]. Moreover, these compounds prevent the accumulation of homocysteine in the brain, in addition to many other organs that are involved in increasing oxidative stress [69]. The etiology of ASD could be a relevant genetic component [70]. Nonetheless, environmental factors can contribute significantly to the disease's evolution [71].

Strengths and Limitations

Accurate quantification of dietary intake in free-living populations is a major challenge in nutritional epidemiology. Moreover, there is a strong debate over the validity of memory-based dietary assessment methods utilized in epidemiological research related to food group consumption and major events of disease [72]. In the present study, to evaluate the food consumption and estimate the nutrient intake, both a FFQ and a 24-hDR were used in a homogeneous sample of Spanish children from the same area and sharing the same socio-cultural habits. Because of its standardized format and the way these questionnaires are administered, they are methods with high performance in terms of cost-effectiveness, which has contributed to their widespread use in large epidemiological cohort studies and also with other designs. However, they have the disadvantage of incorporating systematic errors and biases, which is why procedures are currently being sought to improve the quality of the data collected [73].

This highlights that nutrient intakes variance is usually augmented due to day-to-day variation in individual intake, resulting in misleading estimates of low or high intakes [74]. To avoid the intra-individual variability of the data and obtain an estimate of the population's usual intake distribution, repeated 24-h-DR must be used.

The use of validated tools for the assessment of DPs is limited. It has been suggested that the assessment of DPs, including their consistency and construct validity, should be evaluated over multiple administrations of the same dietary source, different dietary sources, or across various studies [75,76]. In the present study, we used both PCA and clustering analysis for the estimation of DPs. Based on the available evidence, most identified DPs showed good reproducibility, fair relative validity, and good construct validity across different statistical solutions [75].

One of the major limitations of our study is that we focused on a specific population of ASD children living in the southern of Spain. Therefore, our results should be cross-validated in other regions of Spain and other countries. Likewise, the sample of ASD children was very homogenous with regard to cultural and socio-economic aspects; thus, we cannot establish whether different eating patterns would affect nutrient intake adequacy. Finally, we did not attempt to evaluate gastrointestinal symptoms that could affect DPS and nutrient intakes.

5. Conclusions

In the present study, we reported differential DPs between children with ASD and children from the control using both PCA and hierarchical clustering analysis. This highlights high energy and fat consumption and frequently manufactured products with poor nutritional quality and a low intake of vegetables and fruits in ASD children. Likewise, this work adds further support to previous studies identifying inadequate micronutrient intakes for minerals like iron, iodine, and vitamins of group B. Adequate monitoring of the nutritional presence for these nutrients should be assessed and, if necessary, the use of supplements should be introduced into the diet. Hence, it seems relevant to assess the DPs and nutrient intakes in children with ASD to correct eating behavior disorders and rule out nutritional diseases.

Author Contributions: A.R.G.-F., M.G.-C. and J.L.P.-N., contributed to the study conception and study design. M.G.-C. and J.L.P.-N. coordinated all the study. A.R.G.-F., K.F.-R., P.M.-B. and M.J.d.l.T.-A. collected all the data, acquired the behavioral data, and assisted with regulatory responsibilities and carried out the analysis. J.P.-D. and M.J.d.l.T.-A. realized statistical analysis. J.P.-D., M.G.-C. and A.G. were responsible for the interpretation of the data, as well as drafting the manuscript. All authors have read and agreed to the published version of the manuscript.

Funding: This study was supported by the FUNDACIÓ AGRUPACIÓ Àmbit de la Infància, 404 Research Grant INVEST from the Spanish Society of Pediatrics and Red de Salud Materno Infantil (RED SAMID). Á.G. was co-financed by the Research Plan of the Vice-Rectorate of Research and Transfer of the University of Granada, Spain. The funding bodies did not have any role in the design, collection, analyses, or interpretation of data or in writing the manuscript.

Institutional Review Board Statement: The present work is framed within a broader research project, developed by the Pediatric Research Unit of the Pediatric Service of the Reina Sofia University Hospital of Cordoba, entitled "Monitoring of biomarkers of inflammation, oxidative stress, intestinal microbiota, and heavy metals in Autism Spectrum Disorder in childhood." This study was approved by the Ethics Committee of the Reina Sofia University Hospital of Cordoba, Spain, and follows the rules of Law 14/2007 on Biomedical Research and the Organic Law 15/1999, RD 1720/2007 on the protection of personal data as well as international rules for research using samples from human beings. Part of this project's results has been published elsewhere [52,77–79].

Informed Consent Statement: The participants' parents or legal guardians accepted their inclusion in the study, signing the approved protocol. The confidentiality of the data obtained and any personal data used in this study have been kept and respected.

Data Availability Statement: The datasets generated during and/or analyzed during the current study are available from the corresponding author upon reasonable request.

Acknowledgments: The authors would like to thank the children and their parents for their participation in the study. Julio Plaza-Diaz and Angel Gil are part of the UGR Plan Propio de Investigación 2016 Excellence actions: Unit of Excellence on Exercise and Health (UCEES), University of Granada. Julio Plaza-Díaz is supported by a grant to postdoctoral researchers at foreign universities and research centers from the "Fundación Ramón Areces", Madrid, Spain.

Conflicts of Interest: The authors declare no conflict of interest.

References

1. American Psychology Association. *Paraphilic Disorders. Diagnostic and Statistical Manual of Mental Disorders*; American Psychology Association: Washington, DC, USA, 2013; Volume 5, pp. 685–686.
2. Maenner, M.J.; Shaw, K.A.; Baio, J. Prevalence of autism spectrum disorder among children aged 8 years—Autism and developmental disabilities monitoring network, 11 sites, United States, 2016. *MMWR Surveill. Summ.* **2020**, *69*, 1. [CrossRef]
3. Williams, P.G.; Dalrymple, N.; Neal, J. Eating habits of children with autism. *Pediatr. Nurs.* **2000**, *26*, 259.
4. Ranjan, S.; Nasser, J.A. Nutritional status of individuals with autism spectrum disorders: Do we know enough? *Adv. Nutr.* **2015**, *6*, 397–407. [CrossRef] [PubMed]
5. Lázaro, C.P.; Pondé, M.P. Narratives of mothers of children with autism spectrum disorders: Focus on eating behavior. *Trends Psychiatry Psychother.* **2017**, *39*, 4–11. [CrossRef] [PubMed]
6. Ledford, J.R.; Gast, D.L. Feeding problems in children with autism spectrum disorders: A review. *Focus Autism Other Dev. Disabil.* **2006**, *21*, 153–166. [CrossRef]
7. Råstam, M. Eating disturbances in autism spectrum disorders with focus on adolescent and adult years. *Clin. Neuropsychiatry J. Treat. Eval.* **2008**, *5*, 31–42.
8. Brzoska, A.; Kazek, B.; Koziol, K.; Kapinos-Gorczyca, A.; Ferlewicz, M.; Babraj, A.; Makosz-Raczek, A.; Likus, W.; Paprocka, J.; Matusik, P.; et al. Eating Behaviors of Children with Autism-Pilot Study. *Nutrients* **2021**, *13*, 2687. [CrossRef] [PubMed]
9. Schreck, K.A.; Williams, K.; Smith, A.F. A comparison of eating behaviors between children with and without autism. *J. Autism Dev. Disord.* **2004**, *34*, 433–438. [CrossRef] [PubMed]
10. Hubbard, K.L.; Anderson, S.E.; Curtin, C.; Must, A.; Bandini, L.G. A comparison of food refusal related to characteristics of food in children with autism spectrum disorder and typically developing children. *J. Acad. Nutr. Diet.* **2014**, *114*, 1981–1987. [CrossRef] [PubMed]
11. Hyman, S.L.; Levy, S.E.; Myers, S.M. Identification, evaluation, and management of children with autism spectrum disorder. *Pediatrics* **2020**, *145*, e20193447. [CrossRef] [PubMed]
12. Wigham, S.; Rodgers, J.; South, M.; McConachie, H.; Freeston, M. The interplay between sensory processing abnormalities, intolerance of uncertainty, anxiety and restricted and repetitive behaviours in autism spectrum disorder. *J. Autism Dev. Disord.* **2015**, *45*, 943–952. [CrossRef] [PubMed]
13. Geraghty, M.E.; Depasquale, G.M.; Lane, A.E. Nutritional intake and therapies in autism: A spectrum of what we know: Part 1. *ICAN Infant Child Adolesc. Nutr.* **2010**, *2*, 62–69. [CrossRef]
14. Lukens, C.T.; Linscheid, T.R. Development and validation of an inventory to assess mealtime behavior problems in children with autism. *J. Autism Dev. Disord.* **2008**, *38*, 342–352. [CrossRef] [PubMed]
15. Sharp, W.G.; Berry, R.C.; McCracken, C.; Nuhu, N.N.; Marvel, E.; Saulnier, C.A.; Klin, A.; Jones, W.; Jaquess, D.L. Feeding problems and nutrient intake in children with autism spectrum disorders: A meta-analysis and comprehensive review of the literature. *J. Autism Dev. Disord.* **2013**, *43*, 2159–2173. [CrossRef] [PubMed]
16. Baumer, N.; Spence, S.J. Evaluation and management of the child with autism spectrum disorder. *Contin. Lifelong Learn. Neurol.* **2018**, *24*, 248–275. [CrossRef]
17. Bennetto, L.; Kuschner, E.S.; Hyman, S.L. Olfaction and taste processing in autism. *Biol. Psychiatry* **2007**, *62*, 1015–1021. [CrossRef]
18. Bresnahan, M.; Hornig, M.; Schultz, A.F.; Gunnes, N.; Hirtz, D.; Lie, K.K.; Magnus, P.; Reichborn-Kjennerud, T.; Roth, C.; Schjølberg, S. Association of maternal report of infant and toddler gastrointestinal symptoms with autism: Evidence from a prospective birth cohort. *JAMA Psychiatry* **2015**, *72*, 466–474. [CrossRef]
19. Samsam, M.; Ahangari, R.; Naser, S.A. Pathophysiology of autism spectrum disorders: Revisiting gastrointestinal involvement and immune imbalance. *World J. Gastroenterol. WJG* **2014**, *20*, 9942. [CrossRef]

20. Margari, L.; Marzulli, L.; Gabellone, A.; de Giambattista, C. Eating and Mealtime Behaviors in Patients with Autism Spectrum Disorder: Current Perspectives. *Neuropsychiatr Dis. Treat.* **2020**, *16*, 2083–2102. [CrossRef]
21. Canals-Sans, J.; Esteban-Figuerola, P.; Morales-Hidalgo, P.; Arija, V. Do Children with Autism Spectrum Disorders Eat Differently and Less Adequately than Those with Subclinical ASD and Typical Development? EPINED Epidemiological Study. *J. Autism Dev. Disord.* **2021**. [CrossRef]
22. Stepanova, E.; Dowling, S.; Phelps, M.; Findling, R.L. Pharmacotherapy of emotional and behavioral symptoms associated with autism spectrum disorder in children and adolescents. *Dialogues Clin. Neurosci.* **2017**, *19*, 395.
23. DeFilippis, M. The use of complementary alternative medicine in children and adolescents with autism Spectrum disorder. *Psychopharmacol. Bull.* **2018**, *48*, 40. [PubMed]
24. Nath, D. Complementary and alternative medicine in the school-age child with autism. *J. Pediatr. Health Care* **2017**, *31*, 393–397. [CrossRef] [PubMed]
25. Posar, A.; Visconti, P. Complementary and alternative medicine in autism: The question of omega-3. *Pediatr. Ann.* **2016**, *45*, e103–e107. [CrossRef]
26. Hopf, K.P.; Madren, E.; Santianni, K.A. Use and perceived effectiveness of complementary and alternative medicine to treat and manage the symptoms of autism in children: A survey of parents in a community population. *J. Altern. Complement. Med.* **2016**, *22*, 25–32. [CrossRef] [PubMed]
27. Gil-Hernandez, F.; Gomez-Fernandez, A.R.; la Torre-Aguilar, M.J.; Perez-Navero, J.L.; Flores-Rojas, K.; Martin-Borreguero, P.; Gil-Campos, M. Neurotoxicity by mercury is not associated with autism spectrum disorders in Spanish children. *Ital. J. Pediatr.* **2020**, *46*, 19. [CrossRef]
28. Hernandez, M.; Castellet, J.; Narvaiza, J.; Rincón, J.; Ruiz, E.; Sánchez, E.; Sobradillo, B.; Zurimendi, A. *Curvas y Tablas de Crecimiento*; Instituto de Investigación Sobre Crecimiento y Desarrollo; Fundación Faustino Orbegozo: Bilbao, Spain, 2002.
29. Kim, S.H.; Thurm, A.; Shumway, S.; Lord, C. Multisite study of new autism diagnostic interview-revised (ADI-R) algorithms for toddlers and young preschoolers. *J. Autism Dev. Disord.* **2013**, *43*, 1527–1538. [CrossRef]
30. Fernández-Ballart, J.D.; Piñol, J.L.; Zazpe, I.; Corella, D.; Carrasco, P.; Toledo, E.; Perez-Bauer, M.; Martínez-González, M.Á.; Salas-Salvadó, J.; Martín-Moreno, J.M. Relative validity of a semi-quantitative food-frequency questionnaire in an elderly Mediterranean population of Spain. *Br. J. Nutr.* **2010**, *103*, 1808–1816. [CrossRef] [PubMed]
31. Aranceta-Bartrina, J.; Partearroyo, T.; López-Sobaler, A.M.; Ortega, R.M.; Varela-Moreiras, G.; Serra-Majem, L.; Pérez-Rodrigo, C. Updating the Food-Based Dietary Guidelines for the Spanish Population: The Spanish Society of Community Nutrition (SENC) Proposal. *Nutrients* **2019**, *11*, 2675. [CrossRef]
32. EFSA Panel on Dietetic Products, Nutrition and Allergies (NDA). Scientific Opinion on nutrient requirements and dietary intakes of infants and young children in the European Union. *EFSA J.* **2013**, *11*, 3408.
33. Alamri, E.S. Efficacy of gluten-and casein-free diets on autism spectrum disorders in children. *Saudi Med. J.* **2020**, *41*, 1041–1046. [CrossRef]
34. Horvath, A.; Łukasik, J.; Szajewska, H. ω-3 fatty acid supplementation does not affect autism spectrum disorder in children: A systematic review and meta-analysis. *J. Nutr.* **2017**, *147*, 367–376. [CrossRef]
35. Mari-Bauset, S.; Zazpe, I.; Mari-Sanchis, A.; Llopis-Gonzalez, A.; Morales-Suarez-Varela, M. Evidence of the gluten-free and casein-free diet in autism spectrum disorders: A systematic review. *J. Child Neurol.* **2014**, *29*, 1718–1727. [CrossRef]
36. Reissmann, A.; Hauser, J.; Makulska-Gertruda, E.; Tomsa, L.; Lange, K.W. Gluten-free and casein-free diets in the treatment of autism. *Funct. Foods Health Dis.* **2014**, *4*, 349–361. [CrossRef]
37. Emond, A.; Emmett, P.; Steer, C.; Golding, J. Feeding symptoms, dietary patterns, and growth in young children with autism spectrum disorders. *Pediatrics* **2010**, *126*, e337–e342. [CrossRef] [PubMed]
38. Martins, Y.; Young, R.L.; Robson, D.C. Feeding and eating behaviors in children with autism and typically developing children. *J. Autism Dev. Disord.* **2008**, *38*, 1878–1887. [CrossRef] [PubMed]
39. Schmitt, L.; Heiss, C.J.; Campbell, E.E. A comparison of nutrient intake and eating behaviors of boys with and without autism. *Top. Clin. Nutr.* **2008**, *23*, 23–31. [CrossRef]
40. Clark, M.J.; Slavin, J.L. The effect of fiber on satiety and food intake: A systematic review. *J. Am. Coll. Nutr.* **2013**, *32*, 200–211. [CrossRef] [PubMed]
41. Sahan, A.K.; Ozturk, N.; Demir, N.; Karaduman, A.A.; Serel Arslan, S. A Comparative Analysis of Chewing Function and Feeding Behaviors in Children with Autism. *Dysphagia* **2021**. [CrossRef]
42. Madrigal, C.; Soto-Mendez, M.J.; Hernandez-Ruiz, A.; Valero, T.; Avila, J.M.; Ruiz, E.; Villoslada, F.L.; Leis, R.; Martinez de Victoria, E.; Moreno, J.M.; et al. Energy Intake, Macronutrient Profile and Food Sources of Spanish Children Aged One to <10 Years-Results from the EsNuPI Study. *Nutrients* **2020**, *12*, 893. [CrossRef]
43. Partearroyo, T.; Samaniego-Vaesken, M.L.; Ruiz, E.; Aranceta-Bartrina, J.; Gil, A.; Gonzalez-Gross, M.; Ortega, R.M.; Serra-Majem, L.; Varela-Moreiras, G. Current Food Consumption amongst the Spanish ANIBES Study Population. *Nutrients* **2019**, *11*, 2663. [CrossRef]
44. Plaza-Diaz, J.; Molina-Montes, E.; Soto-Mendez, M.J.; Madrigal, C.; Hernandez-Ruiz, A.; Valero, T.; Lara Villoslada, F.; Leis, R.; Martinez de Victoria, E.; Moreno, J.M.; et al. Clustering of Dietary Patterns and Lifestyles Among Spanish Children in the EsNuPI Study (dagger). *Nutrients* **2020**, *12*, 2536. [CrossRef]

45. Samaniego-Vaesken, M.L.; Partearroyo, T.; Valero, T.; Rodriguez, P.; Soto-Mendez, M.J.; Hernandez-Ruiz, A.; Villoslada, F.L.; Leis, R.; Martinez de Victoria, E.; Moreno, J.M.; et al. Carbohydrates, Starch, Total Sugar, Fiber Intakes and Food Sources in Spanish Children Aged One to <10 Years-Results from the EsNuPI Study. *Nutrients* **2020**, *12*, 3171. [CrossRef] [PubMed]
46. Sharp, W.G.; Postorino, V.; McCracken, C.E.; Berry, R.C.; Criado, K.K.; Burrell, T.L.; Scahill, L. Dietary intake, nutrient status, and growth parameters in children with autism spectrum disorder and severe food selectivity: An electronic medical record review. *J. Acad. Nutr. Diet.* **2018**, *118*, 1943–1950. [CrossRef]
47. Tachibana, Y.; Miyazaki, C.; Ota, E.; Mori, R.; Hwang, Y.; Kobayashi, E.; Terasaka, A.; Tang, J.; Kamio, Y. A systematic review and meta-analysis of comprehensive interventions for pre-school children with autism spectrum disorder (ASD). *PLoS ONE* **2017**, *12*, e0186502. [CrossRef] [PubMed]
48. Busdiecker, S.; Castillo, C.; Salas, I. Cambios en los hábitos de alimentación durante la infancia: Una visión antropológica. *Rev. Chil. Pediatr.* **2000**, *71*, 5–11. [CrossRef]
49. Babinska, K.; Celusakova, H.; Belica, I.; Szapuova, Z.; Waczulikova, I.; Nemcsicsova, D.; Tomova, A.; Ostatnikova, D. Gastrointestinal Symptoms and Feeding Problems and Their Associations with Dietary Interventions, Food Supplement Use, and Behavioral Characteristics in a Sample of Children and Adolescents with Autism Spectrum Disorders. *Int. J. Environ. Res. Public Health* **2020**, *17*, 6372. [CrossRef]
50. Kohane, I.S.; McMurry, A.; Weber, G.; MacFadden, D.; Rappaport, L.; Kunkel, L.; Bickel, J.; Wattanasin, N.; Spence, S.; Murphy, S. The co-morbidity burden of children and young adults with autism spectrum disorders. *PLoS ONE* **2012**, *7*, e33224. [CrossRef]
51. Esteban-Figuerola, P.; Canals, J.; Fernandez-Cao, J.C.; Arija Val, V. Differences in food consumption and nutritional intake between children with autism spectrum disorders and typically developing children: A meta-analysis. *Autism* **2019**, *23*, 1079–1095. [CrossRef] [PubMed]
52. Rangel-Huerta, O.D.; Gomez-Fernandez, A.; de la Torre-Aguilar, M.J.; Gil, A.; Perez-Navero, J.L.; Flores-Rojas, K.; Martin-Borreguero, P.; Gil-Campos, M. Metabolic profiling in children with autism spectrum disorder with and without mental regression: Preliminary results from a cross-sectional case-control study. *Metabolomics* **2019**, *15*, 99. [CrossRef]
53. Jory, J. Abnormal fatty acids in Canadian children with autism. *Nutrition* **2016**, *32*, 474–477. [CrossRef]
54. Vancassel, S.; Durand, G.; Barthelemy, C.; Lejeune, B.; Martineau, J.; Guilloteau, D.; Andres, C.; Chalon, S. Plasma fatty acid levels in autistic children. *Prostaglandins Leukot. Essent. Fat. Acids (PLEFA)* **2001**, *65*, 1–7. [CrossRef]
55. Amminger, G.P.; Berger, G.E.; Schafer, M.R.; Klier, C.; Friedrich, M.H.; Feucht, M. Omega-3 fatty acids supplementation in children with autism: A double-blind randomized, placebo-controlled pilot study. *Biol. Psychiatry* **2007**, *61*, 551–553. [CrossRef]
56. Bell, J.G.; Sargent, J.R.; Tocher, D.R.; Dick, J.R. Red blood cell fatty acid compositions in a patient with autistic spectrum disorder: A characteristic abnormality in neurodevelopmental disorders? *Prostaglandins Leukot. Essent. Fat. Acids (PLEFA)* **2000**, *63*, 21–25. [CrossRef]
57. Bozzatello, P.; Brignolo, E.; De Grandi, E.; Bellino, S. Supplementation with Omega-3 Fatty Acids in Psychiatric Disorders: A Review of Literature Data. *J. Clin. Med.* **2016**, *5*, 67. [CrossRef] [PubMed]
58. Das, U. Long-chain polyunsaturated fatty acids in the growth and development of the brain and memory. *Nutrition* **2003**, *19*, 62. [CrossRef]
59. Karhu, E.; Zukerman, R.; Eshraghi, R.S.; Mittal, J.; Deth, R.C.; Castejon, A.M.; Trivedi, M.; Mittal, R.; Eshraghi, A.A. Nutritional interventions for autism spectrum disorder. *Nutr. Rev.* **2020**, *78*, 515–531. [CrossRef] [PubMed]
60. Agostoni, C.; Nobile, M.; Ciappolino, V.; Delvecchio, G.; Tesei, A.; Turolo, S.; Crippa, A.; Mazzocchi, A.; Altamura, C.A.; Brambilla, P. The role of omega-3 fatty acids in developmental psychopathology: A systematic review on early psychosis, autism, and ADHD. *Int. J. Mol. Sci.* **2017**, *18*, 2608. [CrossRef] [PubMed]
61. Cheng, Y.-S.; Tseng, P.-T.; Chen, Y.-W.; Stubbs, B.; Yang, W.-C.; Chen, T.-Y.; Wu, C.-K.; Lin, P.-Y. Supplementation of omega 3 fatty acids may improve hyperactivity, lethargy, and stereotypy in children with autism spectrum disorders: A meta-analysis of randomized controlled trials. *Neuropsychiatr. Dis. Treat.* **2017**, *13*, 2531. [CrossRef] [PubMed]
62. Mazahery, H.; Stonehouse, W.; Delshad, M.; Kruger, M.C.; Conlon, C.A.; Beck, K.L.; Von Hurst, P.R. Relationship between long chain n-3 polyunsaturated fatty acids and autism spectrum disorder: Systematic review and meta-analysis of case-control and randomised controlled trials. *Nutrients* **2017**, *9*, 155. [CrossRef]
63. FAO. *Grasas y Ácidos Grasos en Nutrición Humana Consulta de Expertos*; Organización de las Naciones Unidas para la Alimentación y la Agricultura [FAO] y la Fundación Iberoamericana de Nutrición [FINUT]: Ginebra, Switzerland, 2008; pp. 1–175.
64. Ministry of Environment and Rural and Marine Affairs (MARM) (2008–2021). La Alimentación en España. Ministerio de Agricultura, Pesca y Alimentación, Madrid, España: Madrid. Available online: https://www.mapa.gob.es/es/estadistica/temas/estadisticas-pesqueras/default.aspx (accessed on 1 September 2021).
65. Hyman, S.L.; Stewart, P.A.; Schmidt, B.; Lemcke, N.; Foley, J.T.; Peck, R.; Clemons, T.; Reynolds, A.; Johnson, C.; Handen, B. Nutrient intake from food in children with autism. *Pediatrics* **2012**, *130*, S145–S153. [CrossRef]
66. Malhi, P.; Venkatesh, L.; Bharti, B.; Singhi, P. Feeding problems and nutrient intake in children with and without autism: A comparative study. *Indian J. Pediatr.* **2017**, *84*, 283–288. [CrossRef]
67. Adams, J.B.; Audhya, T.; McDonough-Means, S.; Rubin, R.A.; Quig, D.; Geis, E.; Gehn, E.; Loresto, M.; Mitchell, J.; Atwood, S. Effect of a vitamin/mineral supplement on children and adults with autism. *BMC Pediatr.* **2011**, *11*, 1–30. [CrossRef] [PubMed]
68. Amberg, N.; Laukoter, S.; Hippenmeyer, S. Epigenetic cues modulating the generation of cell-type diversity in the cerebral cortex. *J. Neurochem.* **2019**, *149*, 12–26. [CrossRef] [PubMed]

69. James, S.J.; Melnyk, S.; Jernigan, S.; Cleves, M.A.; Halsted, C.H.; Wong, D.H.; Cutler, P.; Bock, K.; Boris, M.; Bradstreet, J.J. Metabolic endophenotype and related genotypes are associated with oxidative stress in children with autism. *Am. J. Med. Genet. Part B Neuropsychiatr. Genet.* **2006**, *141*, 947–956. [CrossRef] [PubMed]
70. Abrahams, B.S.; Geschwind, D.H. Connecting genes to brain in the autism spectrum disorders. *Arch. Neurol.* **2010**, *67*, 395–399. [CrossRef] [PubMed]
71. Modabbernia, A.; Velthorst, E.; Reichenberg, A. Environmental risk factors for autism: An evidence-based review of systematic reviews and meta-analyses. *Mol. Autism* **2017**, *8*, 1–16. [CrossRef] [PubMed]
72. Archer, E.; Marlow, M.L.; Lavie, C.J. Controversy and debate: Memory-Based Methods Paper 1: The fatal flaws of food frequency questionnaires and other memory-based dietary assessment methods. *J. Clin. Epidemiol.* **2018**, *104*, 113–124. [CrossRef] [PubMed]
73. Golley, R.; Bell, L.; Hendrie, G.A.; Rangan, A.M.; Spence, A.; McNaughton, S.; Carpenter, L.; Allman-Farinelli, M.; de Silva, A.; Gill, T. Validity of short food questionnaire items to measure intake in children and adolescents: A systematic review. *J. Hum. Nutr. Diet.* **2017**, *30*, 36–50. [CrossRef] [PubMed]
74. Mackerras, D.; Rutishauser, I. 24-Hour national dietary survey data: How do we interpret them most effectively? *Public Health Nutr.* **2005**, *8*, 657–665. [CrossRef]
75. Edefonti, V.; De Vito, R.; Dalmartello, M.; Patel, L.; Salvatori, A.; Ferraroni, M. Reproducibility and validity of a posteriori dietary patterns: A systematic review. *Adv. Nutr.* **2020**, *11*, 293–326. [CrossRef]
76. Moeller, S.M.; Reedy, J.; Millen, A.E.; Dixon, L.B.; Newby, P.; Tucker, K.L.; Krebs-Smith, S.M.; Guenther, P.M. Dietary patterns: Challenges and opportunities in dietary patterns research: An Experimental Biology workshop, April 1, 2006. *J. Am. Diet. Assoc.* **2007**, *107*, 1233–1239. [CrossRef]
77. Gomez-Fernandez, A.; de la Torre-Aguilar, M.J.; Gil-Campos, M.; Flores-Rojas, K.; Cruz-Rico, M.D.; Martin-Borreguero, P.; Perez-Navero, J.L. Children With Autism Spectrum Disorder With Regression Exhibit a Different Profile in Plasma Cytokines and Adhesion Molecules Compared to Children Without Such Regression. *Front. Pediatr.* **2018**, *6*, 264. [CrossRef]
78. Plaza-Diaz, J.; Gomez-Fernandez, A.; Chueca, N.; Torre-Aguilar, M.J.; Gil, A.; Perez-Navero, J.L.; Flores-Rojas, K.; Martin-Borreguero, P.; Solis-Urra, P.; Ruiz-Ojeda, F.J.; et al. Autism Spectrum Disorder (ASD) with and without Mental Regression is Associated with Changes in the Fecal Microbiota. *Nutrients* **2019**, *11*, 337. [CrossRef]
79. Martin-Borreguero, P.; Gomez-Fernandez, A.R.; De La Torre-Aguilar, M.J.; Gil-Campos, M.; Flores-Rojas, K.; Perez-Navero, J.L. Children With Autism Spectrum Disorder and Neurodevelopmental Regression Present a Severe Pattern After a Follow-Up at 24 Months. *Front. Psychiatry* **2021**, *12*, 644324. [CrossRef] [PubMed]

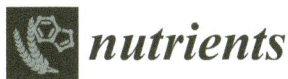

Article

Individual Behavioral Reactions in the Context of Food Sensitivities in Children with Attention-Deficit/Hyperactivity Disorder before and after an Oligoantigenic Diet

Elena Yorgidis †, Lisa Beiner †, Nicola Blazynski †, Katja Schneider-Momm, Hans-Willi Clement, Reinhold Rauh, Eberhard Schulz, Christina Clement *,‡ and Christian Fleischhaker *,‡

Department of Child and Adolescent Psychiatry, Psychotherapy and Psychosomatics, Faculty of Medicine, Medical Center—University of Freiburg, D-79104 Freiburg, Germany; elena.yorgidis@gmx.de (E.Y.); lisa.beiner@uniklinik-freiburg.de (L.B.); n.blazynski@gmail.com (N.B.); katja.schneider-momm@uniklinik-freiburg.de (K.S.-M.); hans-willi.clement@uniklinik-freiburg.de (H.-W.C.); reinhold.rauh@uniklinik-freiburg.de (R.R.); profeberhardschulz@gmx.de (E.S.)
* Correspondence: christina.clement@uniklinik-freiburg.de (C.C.);
  christian.fleischhaker@uniklinik-freiburg.de (C.F.); Tel.: +49-761-270-68620 (C.F.); Fax: +49-761-270-69490 (C.F.)
† The authors contributed equally to this work.
‡ These authors share senior authorship.

Abstract: The influence of food intake on behavior problems of children with Attention-Deficit/Hyperactivity Disorder (ADHD) was already described in the early 20th century. Eliminating food components by using the Oligoantigenic Diet (OD) leads to reduction of ADHD symptoms for more than two-thirds of patients. The aim of our study was to reveal how to identify foods having an impact on ADHD symptomatology. Therefore, 28 children with ADHD participating in this uncontrolled, open trial were examined before and after a restricted elimination diet. They kept a daily 24-h recall nutrition and behavior journal and filled out the abbreviated Conners' scale (ACS) to identify foods which increased ADHD symptoms. The study was completed by 16 children (13 m/3 f). After four weeks of elimination diet the individual food sensitivities were identified in a reintroduction phase. A repetitive increase of ADHD symptoms by at least two points in ACS after food introduction hints at food sensitivity. Twenty-seven food sensitivity reactions were identified. Most of the participants were sensitive to more than one food. Food intolerances could not be identified without preceding OD. The combination of OD and subsequent food challenge appears as a valid method to identify individual food sensitivity in ADHD.

Keywords: adolescents; attention-deficit/hyperactivity disorder; behavior; child; diet; elimination; food intolerance; nutrition; Oligoantigenic Diet

1. Introduction

With a worldwide prevalence of 5.3% among children and adolescents, Attention-Deficit/Hyperactivity Disorder (ADHD) is the most common behavioral disorder [1,2]. ADHD occurs across cultures in about 5% of children and about 2.5% of adults. In children there is a gender related ratio of 2:1 (male: female), [3]. The mechanisms triggering ADHD have not yet been fully identified. Genetic predisposition and pre-, peri- and postnatal environmental influences play a decisive role as do multiple interacting factors [4–6]. Nutrition also plays a role in the development of ADHD [7]. Previous study results have supported the theory that ADHD is an expression of a genetically determined neurodevelopmental disorder. Depending on the degree of severity, the guidelines recommend different treatment options, including parent training, behavioral therapy, pharmacotherapy, and dietary interventions [8–10].

As early as 1922, Shannon noted an increase in restlessness and sleep disorder in children in association with food allergies. After eliminating foods such as tomatoes, eggs

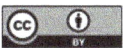

and grains, there was reduction or even disappearance of ADHD symptoms [10]. In 1983, Egger et al. were the first to carry out the Oligoantigenic Diet (OD)—as a dietary diagnostic method to identify food allergies in the field of allergology—in the context of ADHD. Foodstuffs during diet were consciously reduced to very few hypoallergenic foods. The choice of food was initially kept to a minimum. Approved foods were hypoallergenic, mainly including foods which rarely caused adverse reactions. Throughout the OD the ADHD patients showed significant improvements: of 76 participants in this study, 62 children reduced their symptoms. Furthermore, 21 patients no longer met diagnostic criteria for ADHD. Most children responded to two to seven different foods. Re-exposure to the foods caused reappearance or intensified symptoms of ADHD [11]. A study by Pelsser et al. (2009) also showed a reduction in ADHD symptoms after an OD. Here 60% of the participants showed a reduction in symptoms of at least 50% measured with the ADHD Rating Scale [12].

Since then, further studies have shown that nutrition is a strong mediator and/or moderator of ADHD symptoms [8–22]. Dietary interventions in ADHD including elimination diets have shown highly significant effects [13–15,17–22] with effect sizes up to Cohen's d = 5.0 in unblinded studies [7].

Severe dietary interventions such as restricted elimination diets do have a clear impact on daily life and therefore cannot be kept under blinded conditions. In order to minimize the various biases which influence the assessment of ADHD symptoms, Dölp et al. [22] used blinded video ratings to evaluate their primary outcome diagnostic tool, ARS, in the context of dietary intervention. The results showed hardly any difference between blinded and unblinded ratings. Dölp et al. found that OD can lead to symptom reductions in food sensitive children and adolescents with ADHD. After 4 weeks of diet, approximately 60% of the patients showed significant improvement in their condition in ARS [22].

The objective of the present study is to answer the following questions: is it possible to identify foods that intensify typical ADHD symptoms in children by applying OD? Do the participants show different reactions to the same food? Can individual food sensitivities already be identified in a pre-diet phase? Can strong leads to later diagnosed food sensitivities be seen already in the anamnesis?

2. Materials and Methods

The study was approved by the Ethics Committee of Freiburg (application number 111/14) in accordance with the World Medical Association's Declaration of Helsinki. Patients and parents gave written informed consent before participating in the study.

2.1. Participants

The study took place at the Department of Child and Adolescent Psychiatry, Psychotherapy and Psychosomatics of the Medical Center, University of Freiburg. Psychotherapists and general practitioners informed their patients about the study. They were then recruited by study staff. Some participants also became aware of the study via the local press or information on the Internet. Families did not receive any reward for their collaboration in the study.

Interested participants were instructed in detail on the procedure of the study, either in group meetings or individually. ADHD diagnoses were confirmed with Kiddie-SADS-Present and Lifetime Version (K-SADS-PL) [23]. Table 1 shows the characteristics of the participants.

Four of the participants (25%) had a disease at the beginning of the study (rhinitis (n = 2), influenza (n = 1), gastroenteritis (n = 1)).

Table 1. Participants' characteristics.

Included (n)	16 out of 28
Age (means ± SD (range))	9.25 ± 1.73 (7–13)
Gender (m/f)	13/3
Subtypes c/hi/i (n = 28)	16/10/2
Responder (n = 16)	9//6/1
Comorbidity	Dyslexia (F81.0, n = 6)
	Dyscalculia (F81.2, n = 2)
	Oppositional Defiant Disorder (F91.3, F91.8, n = 2)
	Autism (F84.0, n = 2) diagnosed in the course of the study
	Encopresis (F98.1, n = 1)

Subtypes: c: combined type; hi: predominantly hyperactive/impulsive; i: predominantly inattentive.

2.2. Inclusion and Exclusion Criteria

Children and adolescents between the age of 7 and 18 attending at least 2nd grade of a general education school with a confirmed ADHD diagnosis according to the criteria of ICD-10 were included in the study. Children and their parents had to sign for informed consent.

Exclusion criteria were severe concomitant disease, neurological or organic comorbidities which cannot be subjected to dietary intervention. Patients could not participate if there was a lack of compliance either of the parents or children, or a lack of reading or writing skills. Concurrent drug therapy of ADHD or participation in other studies at the same time was not allowed. Children were not to be included when following a special diet (e.g., vegetarian, vegan).

2.3. Measures

The primary outcome was measured using the ADHD rating scale IV (ARS) that is frequently used in ADHD trials [24–34].

2.4. Anamnesis Concerning Food Sensitivity and Allergies in the Beginning

Participants were asked about existing food intolerances, such as allergic reactions to foodstuff or diagnosed food intolerances such as malabsorption or enzyme deficiency.

In the special dietary anamnesis, the children were asked about their preferences and aversions to certain foods.

2.5. Conners' Rating Scale

To assess daily changes of behavior more precisely, the abbreviated Conners' scale (ACS) was used on a daily basis [15,35,36]. In addition to diagnostics, the Conners' scales are important for treatment planning, monitoring, and therapy evaluation. The ACS used here is derived from the long version (105 items), the Conners 3®. This is composed of the items that achieved the highest scores in patients with ADHD and which react very sensitively to therapy effects. Therefore, they are suitable as a short-term follow-up and therapy evaluation [35]. It consists of ten selected items. The ten items are: (1) restless and overactive; (2) excitable impulsive; (3) disturbs other children; (4) fails to finish things—short attention span; (5) constantly fidgeting; (6) inattentive, easily distracted; (7) demands must be met immediately—easily frustrated, (8) cries often and easily; (9) mood changes quickly and drastically (10) temper outbursts, explosive and unpredictable behavior.

Each item was assessed on a 4-point rating scale which resulted in a total score ranging from 0 to 3. With a time requirement of about five minutes, the ACS is a suitable instrument for daily progress monitoring or therapy evaluation. [36].

2.6. Nutrition and Behavior Diary

The nutrition and behavior diary, developed for this study, is based on the allergy diary described by Körner and Schareina [35]. It was kept daily as a 24-h recall protocol by the parents and/or children during the entire study in order to be able to track a temporal and causal relationship between the foods consumed and the occurring ADHD symptoms [34].

Leisure activities that may also affect ACS are also reported e.g., birthday parties, physical training, circus events, and school hiking days.

2.7. Procedure

Initial examination, verifying the ADHD diagnosis, and an assessment of medical health status was followed by a one-week retrospective ADHD rating scale IV [24]. T0 was considered baseline. Figure 1 shows the timeline of the study.

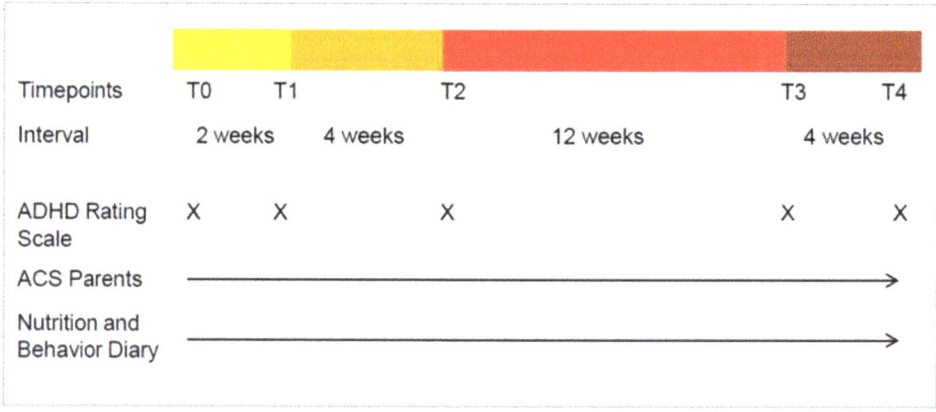

Figure 1. Timescales and measures for each appointment. Yellow bar: pre-diet phase, no change in everyday food intake; Orange bar: diet phase OD; Red bars: food challenge phase, testing the different main food groups. T0: physical examination, Baseline ARS; T1: physical examination, ARS; T2: physical examination, ARS; T3: physical examination, ARS; T4: physical examination, ARS, individual dietary recommendations.

Between T0 and T4, parent ACS and 24-h nutrition and behavior protocols were kept daily. Participants were asked to keep their daily eating habits.

From T1–T2 the children and their families are in a 4-week period of OD. During the diet phase, only a limited selection of hypoallergenic food was allowed to be eaten. The structure of this diet was based on the protocol of Egger et al. and Pelsser et al. [11,14]. Supplementation of vitamins and minerals was advised.

At all time-points, physical examination was kept by a medical professional. At T0, the physical condition and basic neurological findings were additionally recorded.

Throughout the study the families were advised by a nutritionist in order to avoid the risk of malnutrition and to facilitate the implementation of the diet.

All children with an improvement of at least 40% in the ARS total between T1 and T2 were considered to be responders [14].

During T2–T4 the reintroduction of usually consumed foods was proceeded at a time interval of 3–4 days testing each food. ACS questionnaire was completed daily and the nutrition and behavior diary was maintained.

Food sensitivities were defined for foods that showed a repetitive increase in symptoms of at least 2 points on the ACS scale after ingestion compared to the three days before baseline. After identifying the intolerant food in the reintroduction phase, it was assessed whether the intolerant food was consumed before the diet.

2.8. Statistics

The data of 16 participants (out of 28) that completed the whole study was included in statistical analysis.

In cases in which subsamples exceeded five observations, *t*-tests were performed to compare ACS values on the day of reintroduction (dE0), and one, two or three days after reintroduction (dE + 1, dE + 2, dE + 3, etc.) of a particular food to the values one day before reintroduction (dE − 1). All subsamples were too small to apply more complex statistical analyses such as ANOVA with repeated measurements. All statistical analyses were performed with SPSS version 23.0 (IBM Corporation, Armonk, NY, USA).

3. Results

3.1. Participants

16 out of 28 children and adolescents completed the study. The proportion by gender corresponds to the general prevalence of ADHD worldwide. We had 81% male and 19% female participants in our study.

During the diet phase 12 participants either dropped out (*n* = 2) of the study at their own request or were considered non-responders (*n* = 10). None of the participants had medical treatment for ADHD during the whole study (Table 2).

Table 2. Characteristics of dropped out participants.

Dropped out (*n*)	12 out of 28
Age (means ± SD (range))	10.5 ± 1.86 (8–14)
Gender (m/f)	9/3

3.2. ADHD Symptoms According to ARS

The results of this study show that, under careful supervision, children can maintain a 4 weeks OD as documented in the nutrition and health diary. Reductions in ADHD symptoms of 40% or more were seen in 17 participants.

At T0, the 28 ARS parent ratings yielded M = 30.36 and SD = 8.87. Figure 2 shows the individual ARS total score trajectories from T0 to T2.

After 2 weeks (T1) of continuing usual nutrition behavior, parental ARS was not significantly different to T0 (T0: M = 30.36, SD = 8.87; T1: M = 29.54, SD = 9.64; $F(1, 27) < 1$).

From the 28 participants starting the diet, 26 (91.6%) completed. As shown in Figure 2A, after 4 weeks of OD (T2) we observed a significant reduction of ARS total score (T2: M = 15.62, SD = 8.05, $F(1, 25) = 112.34$, $p < 0.0001$). The percentage of improvement observed after the diet, according to the change in ARS total score, was 47.4% on average, ranging from 3.3% to 81.8%. Nine children showed at least 40% symptom reductions in both ARS subscales of inattention and hyperactivity/impulsivity. Thirteen children showed at least a 40% reduction in one subscale. Only three of the participants did not respond in either subscale.

According to Storebø et al. [27] a change of 6.6 points on the ARS is considered as the minimum for a clinically relevant difference. 22 of the 26 participants (84%) showed improvements of between 9 and 27 points between T1 and T2. Three of the 26 participants (11%) showed improvements of between 9 and 13 points between T0 and T1.

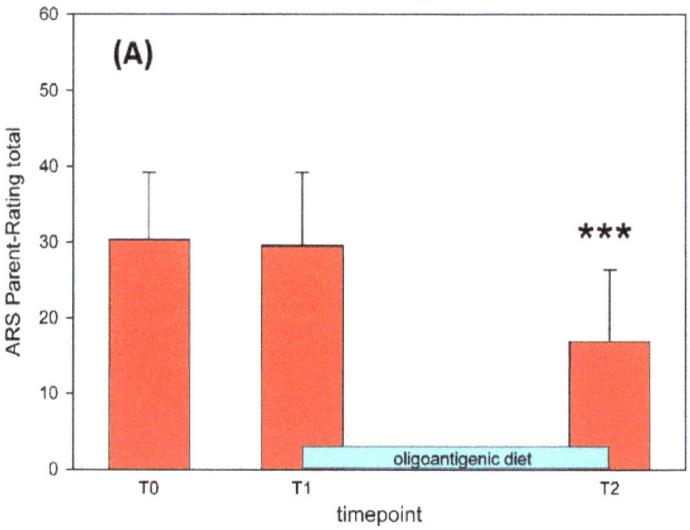

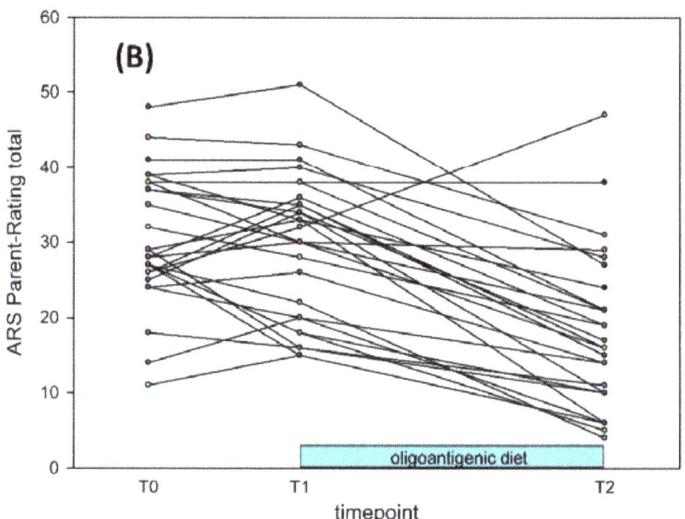

Figure 2. (**A**) Average changes in all participants (*n* = 28) of the ARS scores at each time point (means ± SD), *p* < 0.001 *** (ANOVA with repeated measurements). (**B**) ADHD Rating Scale total scale for all participants in the study. *n* = 28, T0: Baseline, T1: Start of the OD, T2: End of the OD.

3.3. Identified Food Sensitivity

The statistical analysis of the reintroduction phase showed 27 different types of food sensitivity (see Figure 3).

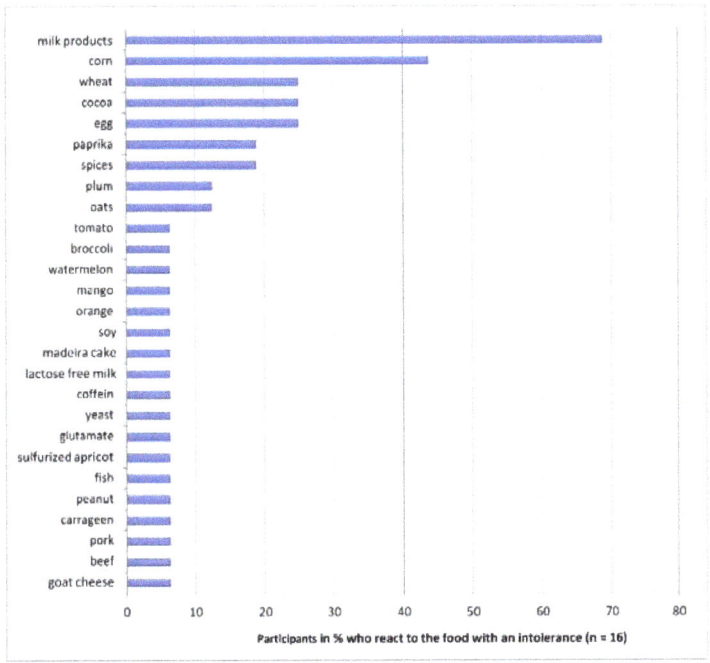

Figure 3. Identified food sensitivities during the study: Percentages of children ($n = 16$) reacting to the respective food with an increase in ADHD symptoms.

3.4. Reactions to Intolerant Food after the OD

Each responder to the OD showed individual food sensitivity, reacting to between 1–10 different foods in the food challenge phase. The three most common detected sensitivities are listed below as examples.

3.4.1. Example 1: Milk Products

The group of dairy consisted of milk, yoghurt, curd cheese, cream, cheese and butter made from cow's milk. Lactose-free products and products made from sheep's or goat's milk were not included.

A total of 68.8% ($n = 11$) of respondents showed a change in ACS after taking dairy products. Among the foods tested, milk products are the ones that most often lead to an increase in ACS levels.

On average, the analysis shows a significant increase in ACS on days dE + 1, dE + 2 and dE + 3 with a sustained effect observed for three days.

Evaluating the milk products, we found two differently reacting groups as shown in Figure 4. Group 1 ($n = 5$) initially responded to the intake of milk products with a decrease in ACS followed by a significant increase in the ACS rating after 1 day. In contrast, group 2 ($n = 6$) showed a significant increase in the ACS rating on the day of consumption of dairy.

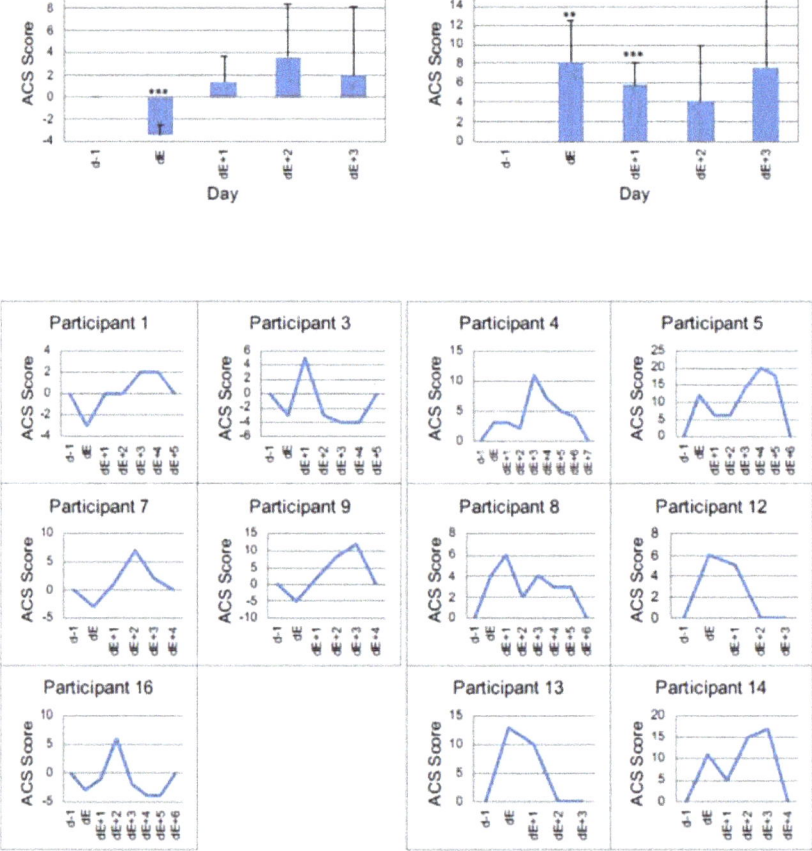

Figure 4. Individual reactions of participants to dairy products, measured by ACS. Group 1 (participants with a decrease of value in ACS at day of reintroduction) vs. Group 2 (participants with an increase of value in ACS at the day of reintroduction) $p < 0.05$ *, $p < 0.01$ **, $p < 0.001$ *** (one sided t-test). dE − 1: day before reintroduction, dE: day of reintroduction, dE + 1: day 1 after reintroduction etc.

Figure 4, Tables 3 and 4 show the daily courses of the mean values as well as the standard deviations of all children in the respective groups. In addition, the individual time courses of each child are displayed.

Table 3. Means and standard deviations of behavioral reactions to dairy products of Group 1 (n = 5).

Day	M	SD	t(4)	p
dE	−3.40	0.89	−8.50	0.001
dE + 1	1.40	2.30	1.36	0.246
dE + 2	3.60	4.83	1.67	0.171
dE + 3	2.00	6.16	0.73	0.508

Table 4. Means and standard deviations of intolerance reactions to dairy products of Group 2 (*n* = 6).

Day	M	SD	t(5)	p
dE	8.17	4.36	4.59	0.006
dE + 1	5.83	2.32	6.17	0.002
dE + 2	4.17	5.74	1.78	0.136
dE + 3	7.67	7.34	2.56	0.051

3.4.2. Example 2: Corn

Figure 5, Tables 5 and 6 show the behavioral reactions to corn.

In total, seven children (43.8%) responded to the intake of products containing corn, as shown in Figure 5.

Group 1 shows a decrease in the ACS value on the day of corn introduction, the largest increase (11 points) on day dE + 1 and a value of 0 on day dE + 3.

Group 2 shows an ACS value increase directly on the day the corn is taken. This is significant on day dE + 1 and dE + 2.

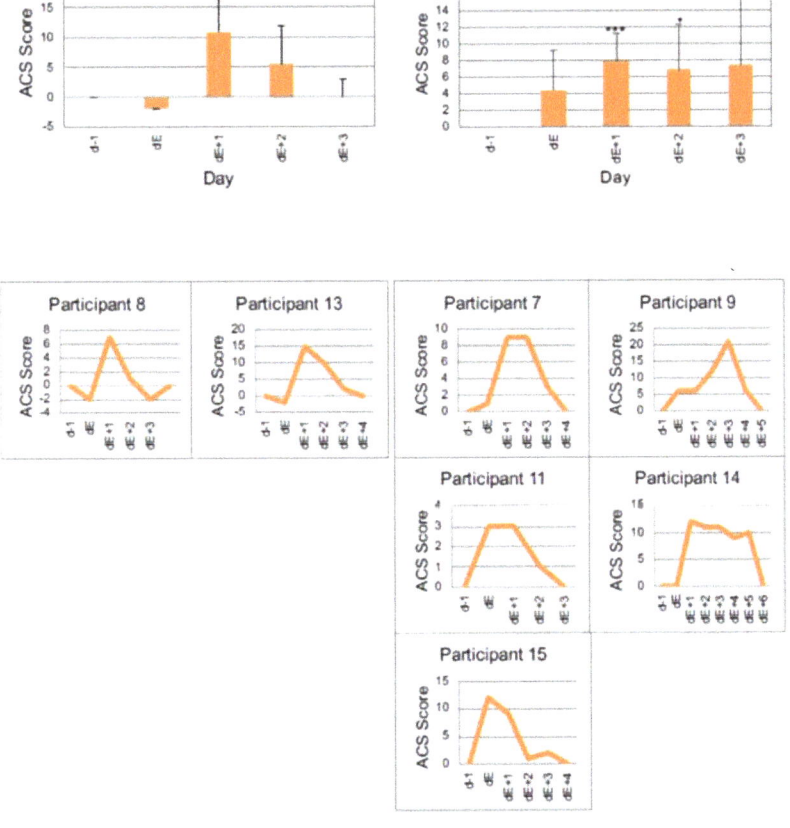

Figure 5. Individual reactions of participants to corn, measured by ACS. Group 1 (participants with a decrease of value in ACS on the day of reintroduction), vs. Group 2 (participants with an increase of value in ACS at the day of reintroduction) $p < 0.05$ *, $p < 0.001$ *** (one-sided *t*-test). dE − 1: day before reintroduction, dE: day of reintroduction, dE + 1: day 1 after reintroduction etc.

Table 5. Means and standard deviations of intolerance reactions to corn of Group 1 (*n* = 2).

Day	M	SD
dE	−2.0	0
dE + 1	11.0	5.66
dE + 2	5.5	6.36
dE + 3	0	2.83

Table 6. Means and standard deviations of behavioral reactions to corn of Group 2 (*n* = 5).

Day	M	SD	t(4)	p
dE	4.40	4.83	2.04	0.111
dE + 1	7.80	3.42	5.10	0.007
dE + 2	6.80	5.40	2.81	0.048
dE + 3	7.40	8.68	1.91	0.129

3.4.3. Example 3: Grain

Figure 6, and Table 7 show the intolerance reaction to grain.

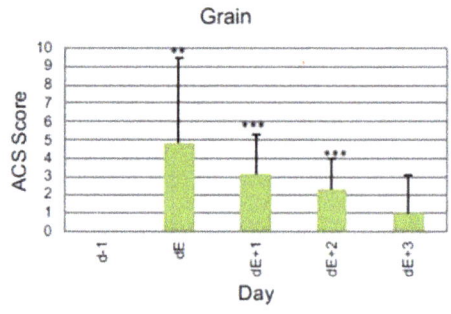

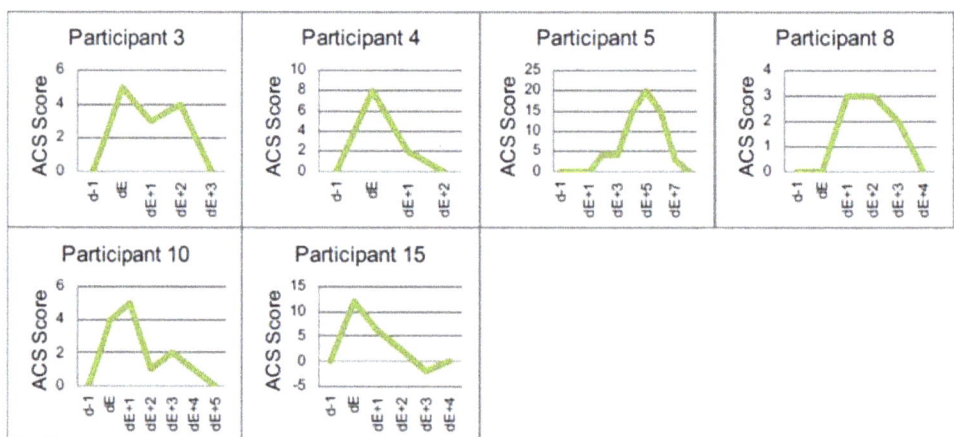

Figure 6. Individual reactions of participants to grain (including oats, wheat and other grain containing gluten) measured by ACS, $p < 0.01$ **, $p < 0.001$ *** (one-sided *t*-test). dE − 1: day before reintroduction, dE: day of reintroduction, dE + 1: day 1 after reintroduction etc.

Table 7. Means and standard deviations of behavioral reactions to grain ($n = 6$).

Day	M	SD	t(5)	p
dE	4.83	4.67	2.54	0.052
dE + 1	3.17	2.14	3.63	0.015
dE + 2	2.33	1.63	3.50	0.017
dE + 3	1.00	2.10	1.17	0.296

For a total of six children (37.5%) the symptoms worsen when eating grain. These include oats, wheat and other grains containing gluten. Corn was excluded.

3.5. Behavioral Reactions to Intolerant Foods before Starting the OD

In the pre-diet phase, 13 out of 16 children consumed several of the observed sensitive foods at the same time. Because of the overlap with the incompatible foods, a reliable prognosis is difficult. In three subjects incompatibilities were observed individually and without overlapping with one another. This was due to the fact that they only reacted to one incompatibility each.

One child showed an increase and decrease in ACS according to the course of the week, so that ACS increased at the weekend without a change in diet (Figure 7A). Overall, none of the children's behavior disturbances can be attributed to a clear food sensitive reaction just on the basis of the data from the pre-diet phase. Two illustrative examples are shown in Figure 7A,B. Figure 7A shows the food sensitivity of one subject before starting the diet. Food sensitivity was safely detected during the reintroduction phase: to milk, cocoa, peanut and corn. Out of four intolerant foods, three were consumed at different timepoints in the pre-diet phase as shown below.

Looking at the individual foods, milk shows an average decrease in ACS within the first 24 h after consuming by −1.67. In the following days there is an increase in ACS compared to the value before the intake (<24 h = −0.67; 24–48 h = +0.67; 48–72 h= +1).

When cocoa is consumed, an immediate increase in ACS is only notable on day 10 (+2). On day 13 there is a delayed increase the next day (+1). The remaining days (day 3, day 6–8) are inconspicuous, with an average increase of 0.5 in the first 24 h (<24 h = 0.5; 24–48 h = −0.5; 48–72 h= −0.5).

Corn was consumed only in small amounts. On day 4, most corn was consumed in the form of popcorn, with a delayed increase of ACS the next day (+3). (<24 h = −0.67; 24–48 h = +1; 48–72 h= −2).

Due to the weak fluctuations, no clear statement is possible. Overall, possible changes in ADHD symptoms due to intolerant foods overlap, which makes a reliable prognosis of individual food sensitivity almost impossible.

Figure 7B shows the reactions of another participant. Food sensitivities safely detected during the reintroduction phase were to bell pepper and wheat. Wheat was supplied daily in the form of baked goods (bread). On average, there was a mean decrease in ACS in the days after ingestion compared to the initial value (<24 h = −0.75; 24–48 h = 0; 48–72 h = −0.75).

Bell peppers were eaten as spice powder (day 3) or raw (day 12). There is a small increase in ACS (+2) on the respective days, but day 12, when raw paprika was eaten, is particularly noteworthy with an increase from +3 to 15 (<24 h = +2; 24–48 h = 0; 48–72 h = +0.5).

It is also noticeable that on days with physical activity (soccer training, swimming training) ACS is relatively low (day 1, 2, 5) or decreased compared to the previous day (day 8). One reason for an increase in ACS could be that subject in 7B had a friend visiting him on day 6 and a birthday party on day 7.

The overlay of food makes a reliable prognosis difficult. In addition, there are fluctuations that may be related to special events in everyday life, which makes it difficult to identify possibly ADHD-promoting foods.

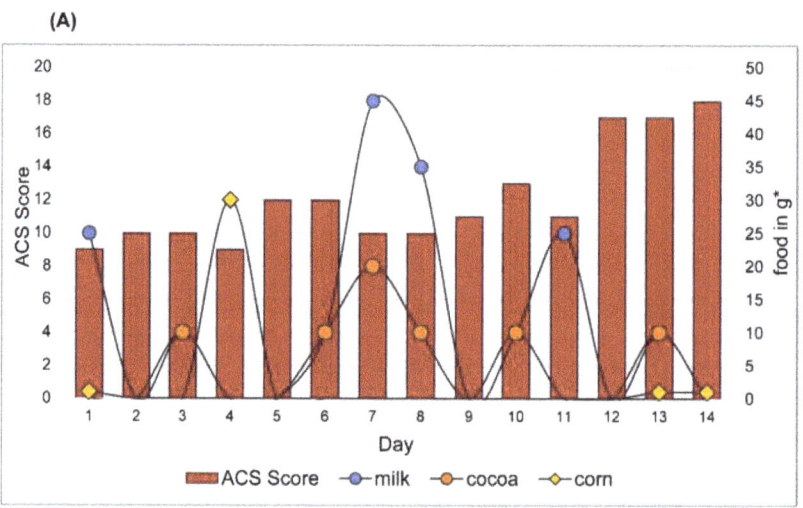

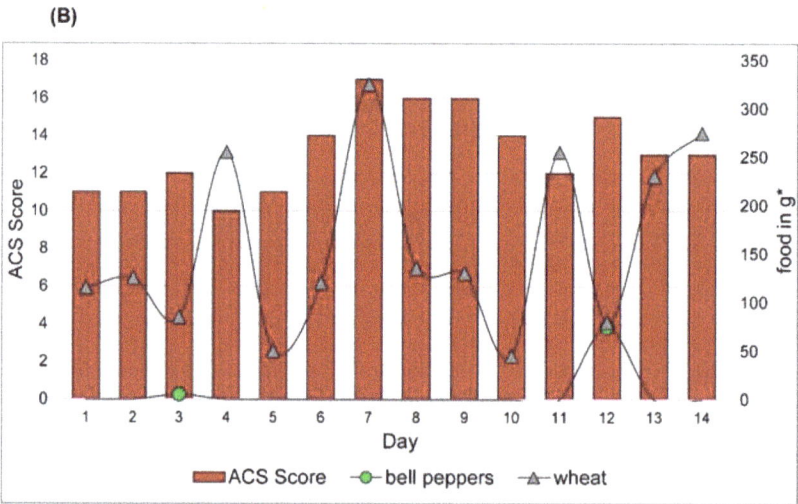

Figure 7. (**A**) Food sensitivity of participant 1. Reactions to different foods in the pre-diet phase. Food sensitivities safely detected during the reintroduction phase: milk, cocoa, peanut and corn. Peanuts are not mentioned because they were not eaten in the pre-diet phase. (**B**) Food sensitivity of participant 2. Reactions to different foods in the pre-diet phase. Food sensitivities safely detected during the reintroduction phase: bell peppers and wheat. ACS value declared by parents, displayed in red bars on the left axis. Amount of intolerable food consumed in grams * shown in lines on the right axis. * estimated amount.

3.6. Anamnestic Intolerance Prior to OD and Observed Sensitivity during Food Reintroduction

In an initial anamnesis, the children were asked about their eating habits. In addition to "likes" and "dislikes," they were also asked about suspected sensitivity as a possible trigger of ADHD. Of the 16 subjects, eleven (68.8%) did not match the information in the anamnesis questionnaire with the sensitivities found later. Of the 16 subjects, there is a match between a favorite food (eggs) and a sensitivity only in one participant (6.25%). One presented (6.25%) a correspondence of a dislike (fish) with an incompatible food. In three of the 16 subjects (18.75%) the suspicion was confirmed. The questionable foods are milk (2) and soy (1). In all three participants, physical symptoms in addition to ADHD symptoms occurred after consuming these foods.

4. Discussion

A main aspect of the study is to show that OD is a useful method to find out if there are food related changes of ADHD symptoms in children. Furthermore, our study is the first to investigate the individual behavioral responses on different foods related to ADHD symptoms.

Pelsser recommends that a change in diet should be considered in all children with ADHD, as Pelsser's study showed a significant effect in children with ADHD and ODD of the elimination diet. This requires medical supervision and parental cooperation when following this restrictive elimination diet [14]. In a previous study we could also show the positive effects of OD in children with ADHD [22].

Before starting the diet, it is not obvious if children react to food, and when they do so, what kind of foodstuff result in an increase of ADHD symptoms. Children included in this study did react after 4 weeks of diet. The participants showed individual food sensitivity concerning type of food, intensity or pattern of reactivity. In all patients, ADHD symptoms were intensified by various foods during the food challenge after OD.

After detecting food related ADHD symptoms by OD, it is important to find out, by reintroduction, to what kind of food the children are sensitive. In our small sample we could demonstrate 27 different foods which increased the symptoms of ADHD in our participants.

Comparing this study with previous studies on the OD by Egger et al., a concordance of frequency of intolerance more often regarding milk products can be shown. Cow's milk sensitivity occurred in 64% of the cases in Egger and Carter, in 60% of the cases in Hiedl, and in our current study in 68% of the cases. From this, one can conclude that the most common food intolerance that leads to an increase in ADHD symptoms is cow's milk. However, not all of the food sensitive children did react to milk, so there should never be a general recommendation to avoid milk in the context of ADHD. In all four studies, wheat and grains in general could be detected as common provoking foods. Egg was also more often on the list of intolerant foods in all studies. [11,13,14,16,37,38], but only individual dietary recommendations should be given in the context of the individually detected food sensitivity.

The study also shows that almost every participant experienced an increase of far more than two points in ACS after the food challenge. The amount and type of reaction were individually different. The strongest reaction was seen in one subject after taking paprika. There was an immediate increase in ADHD symptoms by 25 points as measured by ACS.

It could not be shown that a connection between certain foods and behavior can already be established during the pre-diet phase by evaluating the food and behavior diary. The pre-diet phase should, however, continue to be at the forefront when carrying out an OD to observe usual eating habits and to train the protocoling. It is also useful to have a pre-diet control protocol in order to test whether the change in daily life when focusing on nutrition and behavior of the child does influence ADHD symptoms or not.

An OD with subsequent reintroduction can be the most useful diagnostic tool to identify individual food sensitivity in connection with ADHD. Because every participant reacted very individually to different foods, there must be an individual dietary recommendations for each individual child.

Several possible different pathomechanisms are noted to cause an increase in symptoms. Most children (70%) reacted to milk products. Of these, 73% did not react to dairy products which were free of lactose. This leads to a hypothesis that the pathomechanism of lactose intolerance could be connected to ADHD symptoms. In a previous study from

Edreffy et al. [39], the differences in oligosaccharide metabolism between ADHD and healthy controls were described. This study supports the hypothesis that carbohydrate metabolism differs in ADHD subjects compared to control. Alabaf et al. [40] investigated physical health in children with a neurodevelopmental disorder on the basis of the database of The Children and Adolescent Twin Study in Sweden (CATSS). Their results showed that children 9–12 years of age diagnosed with ADHD suffered more than twice as often from lactose intolerance as the age-matched total population. The occurrence of celiac disease was also described to be higher in patients with ADHD. The prevalence of celiac disease increased significantly in patients with ADHD and comorbidity such as autism spectrum disorder and learning disorder.

We found ADHD related symptoms worsening in children after the consumption of different grains. This could indicate probable digestive problems in the context of different grains. Niederhofer et al. [41] reported an overrepresentation of celiac disease, identified by measuring the celiac specific antibodies anti-gliadin and anti-endomysium in patients with ADHD. Ten out of 67 patients with ADHD were diagnosed with celiac disease. A significant improvement of ADHD symptoms under gluten-free diet was observed by patients and parents. In our study, we also found remission of ADHD symptoms in grain sensitive children after three days of grain-elimination during the food reintroduction.

"Brain-gut axis" and "microbiome" have also been shown to be related to mental disorders [42,43]. Though the microbiome in humans shows a high interpersonal variation, its composition is influenced by geography, culture, and diet [44,45]. The type of nutrition plays a decisive role in the composition of the microbiome. Despite the evidence that abnormal development of the intestinal microbiome has long-term implications on host health, the causal contributions of abnormal intestinal microbiome variations to disease states have yet to be elucidated [45].

One can therefore consider whether there is a complicated mechanism behind ADHD symptoms in relation to food intake. The microbiome can be regarded as a trigger or amplifier of ADHD symptoms [43]. Kumperscak et al. found improvements in children´s behavior after three months probiotic treatment with "*Lactobacillus rhamnosus*" [46]. A randomized controlled trial published in 2016 showed a significant improvement in ADHD symptoms in children with autism after supplementation of "Lactobacillus Plantarum PS128" [47]. These results reinforce the hypothesis of microbial influence on ADHD symptoms.

Pelsser investigated the immunological response comparing allergic and non-allergic reactions in food intolerances and food allergies in children with ADHD. IgE is implicated in typical food allergies. If reactions to foods are not mediated by IgE, the assessment of IgG levels might be useful, when considering the aim of establishing a relation between foods and ADHD. According to this theory, eating foods that induce high IgG levels would lead to a substantial behavioral relapse whereas eating foodstuff that induces low IgG levels would not. The results did not support this hypothesis [14].

This suggests that food sensitivities in ADHD are not necessarily allergic reactions. However, a cell-mediated allergic reaction has not been investigated and therefore cannot be excluded. A pilot study from Dieterich et al. [48] could identify inflammatory processes in the gut reflected in inflammation-related intolerance reactions to foods, without showing a systemic inflammation in blood parameters. Food intolerances relate to high interferon IFN-γ concentrations in different gut regions. Gut mediated reactions to food intolerances showed differences to inflammation parameters in food allergy. In different gut regions, they found an increase of IFN-γ which might result from an unspecific immune response to an intestinal dysbiosis in the intestine and to a release of micro-biotic peptides as described by Farin et al. [49]. This might explain our results concerning the individual reactions to intolerant foods in food reintroduction. We found different intensities of reactions and individual time-courses to recovery. This might be related to a highly individual gut microbiome and subsequently its metabolites, which can stimulate local inflammatory processes in the gut.

This supports the theory that the composition of gut microbiome plays an important role in this context.

Whatever mechanisms a dietary intervention relies on, Stevenson et al. [50] pointed out in their research review form 2014 that a restricted elimination diet might be beneficial for ADHD symptoms in children and adults.

Limitations and Future Directions

The evaluation of the daily behavior could, besides dietary intervention, also be impacted by various factors such as social interactions or physical health.

For the assessment of ADHD symptoms, they must occur in at least two contexts (usually at home and at school). Unfortunately, teacher´s ratings could not be collected in total. This is a clear limitation of the study.

The study was open, non-randomized, without a control group and without blinding the diet. Focusing on behavior and eating habits while implementing serious changes in daily life might lead to a remarkable bias in parent's ratings. To corroborate these preliminary findings, an extension of the study with a larger number of subjects would be important to confirm the effects already observed.

Children had to control their eating behavior by themselves. Whether children always provided their information on food consumption truthfully is not guaranteed. Although the importance of correct information for the diary was clearly explained, there certainly were undocumented dietary violations.

5. Conclusions

The European treatment guidelines on ADHD recommend that restricted elimination diets may be beneficial for children with ADHD and with a history of adverse reactions to food. However, our data indicate that there are many ADHD children without a history of adverse reaction to food that may profit from OD and subsequent identification of highly individual food sensitivity.

In summary of the available results, Oligoantigenic Diet seems to be a useful tool to identify food sensitive ADHD patients. Subsequently, detected individual food sensitivities leading to individualized dietary recommendations are useful as an additional option to the existing multimodal therapy concept.

Author Contributions: E.Y., L.B., N.B., C.C., H.-W.C., C.F. contributed to the literature search, E.Y., L.B., N.B., K.S.-M., H.-W.C., R.R., E.S., C.C., C.F. to the methodology, E.Y., L.B., N.B., H.-W.C., R.R., E.S., C.C., C.F. the interpretation of the data and E.Y., L.B., N.B., H.-W.C., R.R., E.S., C.C., C.F. to the writing of the manuscript. All authors had full access to the data. All authors have read and agreed to the published version of the manuscript.

Funding: This research received no external funding.

Institutional Review Board Statement: The study was approved by the local ethics committee (application number 111/14) in accordance with the World Medical Association's Declaration of Helsinki.

Informed Consent Statement: Informed consent and assent were obtained for all participants involved in the study.

Data Availability Statement: The data are not publicly available according to description of confidentiality and data sharing procedures described in the study's informed consent and assent documents.

Conflicts of Interest: The authors declare no conflict of interest.

References

1. Polanczyk, G.; de Lima, M.S.; Horta, B.L.; Biederman, J.; Rohde, L.A. The Worldwide Prevalence of ADHD: A Systematic Review and Metaregression Analysis. *Am. J. Psychiatry* **2007**, *164*, 942–948. [CrossRef]
2. Sayal, K.; Prasad, V.; Daley, D.; Ford, T.; Coghill, D. ADHD in Children and Young People: Prevalence, Care Pathways, and Service Provision. *Lancet Psychiatry* **2018**, *5*, 175–186. [CrossRef]

3. Taylor, E.; Sergeant, J.; Asherson, P.; Banaschewski, T.; Buitelaar, J.; Coghill, D.; Danckaerts, M.; Rothenberger, A.; Sonuga-Barke, E.; Steinhausen, H.-C.; et al. European Clinical Guidelines for Hyperkinetic Disorder ? First Upgrade. *Eur. Child Adolesc. Psychiatry* **2004**, *13*, i7–i30. [CrossRef]
4. Faraone, S.V.; Perlis, R.H.; Doyle, A.E.; Smoller, J.W.; Goralnick, J.J.; Holmgren, M.A.; Sklar, P. Molecular Genetics of Attention-Deficit/Hyperactivity Disorder. *Biol. Psychiatry* **2005**, *57*, 1313–1323. [CrossRef] [PubMed]
5. Khan, S.A.; Faraone, S.V. The Genetics of ADHD: A Literature Review of 2005. *Curr. Psychiatry Rep.* **2006**, *8*, 393–397. [CrossRef] [PubMed]
6. Gillis, J.J.; Gilger, J.W.; Pennington, B.F.; DeFries, J.C. Attention Deficit Disorder in Reading-Disabled Twins: Evidence for Ge-netic Etiology. *J. Abnorm. Child Psychol.* **1992**, *20*, 303–315. [CrossRef]
7. Sonuga-Barke, E.J.; Brandeis, D.; Cortese, S.; Daley, D.; Ferrin, M.; Holtmann, M.; Stevenson, J.; Danckaerts, M.; Van Der Oord, S.; Döpfner, M.; et al. Nonpharmacological Interventions for ADHD: Systematic Review and Meta-Analyses of Randomized Controlled Trials of Dietary and Psychological Treatments. *Am. J. Psychiatry* **2013**, *170*, 275–289. [CrossRef]
8. American Academy of Pediatrics. Wolraich ML, Hagan JF, Allan C, et al; Subcommittee on Children and Adolescents with Attention-Deficit/Hyperactive Disorder. Clinical Practice Guideline for the Diagnosis, Evaluation, and Treatment of Attention-Deficit/Hyperactivity Disorder in Children and Adolescents. *Pediatrics* **2020**, *145*, e20193997. [CrossRef]
9. Sharma, A.; Couture, J. A Review of the Pathophysiology, Etiology, and Treatment of Attention-Deficit Hyperactivity Disorder (ADHD). *Ann. Pharmacother.* **2014**, *48*, 209–225. [CrossRef] [PubMed]
10. Shannon, W.R. Neuropathic Manifestations in Infants and Children as a Result of Anaphylactic Reaction to Foods Contained in Their Dietary. *Arch. Pediatr. Adolesc. Med.* **1922**, *24*, 89–94. [CrossRef]
11. Egger, J.; Graham, P.; Carter, C.; Gumley, D.; Soothill, J. Controlled Trial of Oligoantigenic Treatment in the HYPERKINETIC SYNDROME. *Lancet* **1985**, *325*, 540–545. [CrossRef]
12. Pelsser, L.; Frankena, K.; Toorman, J.; Savelkoul, H.F.J.; Pereira, R.R.; Buitelaar, J.K. A Randomised Controlled Trial into the Effects of Food on ADHD. *Eur. Child Adolesc. Psychiatry* **2008**, *18*, 12–19. [CrossRef] [PubMed]
13. Pelsser, L.M.; Frankena, K.; Buitelaar, J.K.; Rommelse, N.N. Effects of Food on Physical and Sleep Complaints in Children with ADHD: A Randomised Controlled Pilot Study. *Eur. J. Nucl. Med. Mol. Imaging* **2010**, *169*, 1129–1138. [CrossRef] [PubMed]
14. Pelsser, L.; Frankena, K.; Toorman, J.; Savelkoul, H.F.; Dubois, E.A.; Pereira, R.R.; Haagen, A.T.; Rommelse, N.N.; Buitelaar, J.K. Effects of a Restricted Elimination Diet on the Behaviour of Children with Attention-Deficit Hyperactivity Disorder (INCA study): A Randomised Controlled Trial. *Lancet* **2011**, *377*, 494–503. [CrossRef]
15. Kaplan, B.J.; McNicol, J.; Conte, A.R.; Moghadam, H.K. Dietary replacement in preschool-aged hyperactive boys. *Pediatrics* **1989**, *83*, 7–17. [PubMed]
16. Carter, C.M.; Urbanowicz, M.; Hemsley, R.; Mantilla, L.; Strobel, S.; Graham, P.J.; Taylor, E. Effects of a Few Food Diet in Attention Deficit Disorder. *Arch. Dis. Child.* **1993**, *69*, 564–568. [CrossRef]
17. McCann, D.; Barrett, A.; Cooper, A.; Crumpler, D.; Dalen, L.; Grimshaw, K.; Kitchin, E.; Lok, K.Y.-W.; Porteous, L.; Prince, E.; et al. Food Additives and Hyperactive Behaviour in 3-Year-Old and 8/9-Year-Old Children in the Community: A Randomised, Double-Blinded, Placebo-Controlled Trial. *Lancet* **2007**, *370*, 1560–1567. [CrossRef]
18. Boris, M.; Mandel, F.S. Foods and Additives are Common Causes of the Attention Deficit Hyperactive Disorder in Children. *Ann. Allergy* **1994**, *72*, 462–468.
19. Rytter, M.J.H.; Andersen, L.B.B.; Houmann, T.; Bilenberg, N.; Hvolby, A.; Mølgaard, C.; Michaelsen, K.F.; Lauritzen, L. Diet in the Treatment of ADHD in Children—A Systematic Review of the Literature. *Nord. J. Psychiatry* **2014**, *69*, 1–18. [CrossRef]
20. Hill, P. Current Topic: An Auditable Protocol for Treating Attention Deficit/Hyperactivity Disorder. *Arch. Dis. Child.* **2001**, *84*, 404–409. [CrossRef]
21. Pelsser, L.; Frankena, K.; Toorman, J.; Pereira, R.R. Diet and ADHD, Reviewing the Evidence: A Systematic Review of Meta-Analyses of Double-Blind Placebo-Controlled Trials Evaluating the Efficacy of Diet Interventions on the Behavior of Children with ADHD. *PLoS ONE* **2017**, *12*, e0169277. [CrossRef] [PubMed]
22. Dölp, A.; Schneider-Momm, K.; Heiser, P.; Clement, C.; Rauh, R.; Clement, H.-W.; Schulz, E.; Fleischhaker, C. Oligoantigenic Diet Improves Children's ADHD Rating Scale Scores Reliably in Added Video-Rating. *Front. Psychiatry* **2020**, *11*, 730. [CrossRef]
23. Chambers, W.J.; Puig-Antich, J.; Hirsch, M.; Paez, P.; Ambrosini, P.J.; Tabrizi, M.A.; Davies, M. The Assessment of Affective Dis-Orders in Children and Adolescents by Semistructured Interview. Test-Retest Reliability of the Schedule for Affective Disorders and Schizophrenia for School-Age Children, Present Episode Version. *Arch. Gen. Psychiatry* **1985**, *42*, 696–702. [CrossRef] [PubMed]
24. Dupaul, G.J. Parent and Teacher Ratings of ADHD Symptoms: Psychometric Properties in a Community-Based Sample. *J. Clin. Child Psychol.* **1991**, *20*, 245–253. [CrossRef]
25. Dupaul, G.J.; Reid, R.; Anastopoulos, A.D.; Lambert, M.C.; Watkins, M.W.; Power, T.J. Parent and Teacher Ratings of Attention-Deficit/Hyperactivity Disorder Symptoms: Factor Structure and Normative Data. *Psychol. Assess.* **2016**, *28*, 214–225. [CrossRef]

26. Anastopoulos, A.D.; Beal, K.K.; Reid, R.J.; Reid, R.; Power, T.J.; Dupaul, G.J. Impact of Child and Informant Gender on Parent and Teacher Ratings of Attention-Deficit/Hyperactivity Disorder. *Psychol. Assess.* **2018**, *30*, 1390–1394. [CrossRef]
27. Storebø, O.J.; Ramstad, E.; Krogh, H.B.; Nilausen, T.D.; Skoog, M.; Holmskov, M.; Rosendal, S.; Groth, C.; Magnusson, F.L.; Moreira-Maia, C.R.; et al. Methylphenidate for Children and Adolescents with Attention Deficit Hyperactivity Disorder (ADHD). *Cochrane Database Syst. Rev.* **2015**, CD009885. [CrossRef] [PubMed]
28. Mercier, C.; Roche, S.; Gaillard, S.; Kassai, B.; Arzimanoglou, A.; Herbillon, V.; Roy, P.; Rheims, S. Partial Validation of a French Version of the ADHD-Rating Scale IV on a French Population of Children with ADHD and Epilepsy. Factorial Structure, Reliability, and Responsiveness. *Epilepsy Behav.* **2016**, *58*, 1–6. [CrossRef]
29. Zhang, S.; Faries, D.; Vowles, M.; Michelson, D. ADHD Rating Scale IV: Psychometric Properties from a Multinational Study as Clinician-Administered Instrument. *Int. J. Methods Psychiatr. Res.* **2005**, *14*, 186–201. [CrossRef]
30. Alexandre, J.L.; Lange, A.-M.; Bilenberg, N.; Gorrissen, A.M.; Søbye, N.; Lambek, R. The ADHD Rating Scale-IV Preschool Version: Factor Structure, Reliability, Validity, and Standardisation in a Danish Community Sample. *Res. Dev. Disabil.* **2018**, *78*, 125–135. [CrossRef]
31. Richarte, V.; Corrales, M.; Pozuelo, M.; Serra-Pla, J.; Ibáñez, P.; Calvo, E.; Corominas, M.; Bosch, R.; Casas, M.; Ramos-Quiroga, J.A. Spanish Validation of the Adult Attention Deficit/Hyperactivity Disorder Rating Scale (ADHD-RS): Relevance of clinical subtypes. *Rev. Psiquiatr. Salud Ment.* **2017**, *10*, 185–191. [CrossRef]
32. Wittchen, H.-U.; Zaudig, M.; Fydrich, T. SKID Strukturiertes Klinisches Interview für DSM-IV. Achse I und II. Göttingen: Hogrefe. Zeitschrift für klinische Psychologie und Psychotherapie. 1999. Available online: https://econtent.hogrefe.com/doi/10.1026//0084-5345.28.1.68 (accessed on 27 July 2021).
33. DuPaul, G.J.; Power, T.J.; Anastopoulos, A.D.; Reid, R. *ADHD Rating Scale—IV: Checklists, Norms, and Clinical Interpretation*; Guilford Press: New York, NY, USA, 1998; pp. 1–80.
34. Conners, C.K.; Goyette, C.H.; Southwick, D.A.; Lees, J.M.; Andrulonis, P.A. Food additives and hyperkinesis: A controlled double-blind experiment. *Pediatrics* **1976**, *58*, 154–166.
35. Koerner, U.; Schareina, A. Nahrungsmittelallergien und -Unverträglichkeiten. In *Diagnostik, Therapie und Beratung*; Haug: Stuttgart, Germany, 2010.
36. Lidzba, K.; Christiansen, H.; Drechsler, R. *Conners 3: Conners Skalen zur Aufmerksamkeit und Verhalten-3: Deutschsprachige Adaptation der Conners 3rd Edition (Conners 3) von C. Keith Conners: Manual (K. Conners, Hrsg.)*; Hans Huber: Bern, Switzerland, 2013.
37. Pelsser, L.M.; Van Steijn, D.J.; Frankena, K.; Toorman, J.; Buitelaar, J.K.; Rommelse, N.N. A Randomized Controlled Pilot Study into the Effects of a Restricted Elimination Diet on Family Structure in Families with ADHD and ODD. *Child. Adolesc. Ment. Health* **2012**, *18*, 39–45. [CrossRef] [PubMed]
38. Hiedl, S. *Duodenale VIP-Rezeptoren in der Dünndarmmukosa bei Kindern mit Nahrungsmittelinduziertem Hyperkinetischen Syndrom. Zur Erlangung des Medizinischen Doktorgrades*; Ludwig-Maximilians-Universität München: München, Germany, 2004.
39. Endreffy, I.; Bjørklund, G.; Urbina, M.A.; Chirumbolo, S.; Doşa, M.D.; Dicső, F. High Levels of Glycosaminoglycans in the Urines of Children with Attention-Deficit/Hyperactivity Disorder (ADHD). *J. Mol. Neurosci.* **2020**, *70*, 1018–1025. [CrossRef] [PubMed]
40. Alabaf, S.; Gillberg, C.; Lundström, S.; Lichtenstein, P.; Kerekes, N.; Rastam, M.; Anckarsäter, H. Physical Health in Children with Neurodevelopmental Disorders. *J. Autism Dev. Disord.* **2019**, *49*, 83–95. [CrossRef]
41. Niederhofer, H. Association of Attention-Deficit/Hyperactivity Disorder and Celiac Disease: A Brief Report. *Prim. Care Companion CNS Disord.* **2011**, *13*, e1–e3. [CrossRef] [PubMed]
42. Aarts, E.; Ederveen, T.; Naaijen, J.; Zwiers, M.P.; Boekhorst, J.; Timmerman, H.M.; Smeekens, S.P.; Netea, M.G.; Buitelaar, J.K.; Franke, B.; et al. Gut Microbiome in ADHD and Its Relation to Neural Reward Anticipation. *PLoS ONE* **2017**, *12*, e0183509. [CrossRef]
43. Hiergeist, A.; Gessner, J.; Gessner, A. Current Limitations for the Assessment of the Role of the Gut Microbiome for Attention Deficit Hyperactivity Disorder (ADHD). *Front. Psychiatry* **2020**, *11*, 623. [CrossRef]
44. Schink, M.; Konturek, P.C.; Tietz, E.; Dieterich, W.; Pinzer, T.C.; Wirtz, S.; Neurath, M.F.; Zopf, Y. Microbial Patterns in Patients with Histamine Intolerance. *J. Physiol. Pharmacol.* **2018**, *69*, 579–593.
45. Barko, P.; McMichael, M.; Swanson, K.; Williams, D. The Gastrointestinal Microbiome: A Review. *J. Vet. Intern. Med.* **2017**, *32*, 9–25. [CrossRef] [PubMed]
46. Kumperscak, H.G.; Gricar, A.; Ülen, I.; Micetic-Turk, D. A Pilot Randomized Control Trial with the Probiotic Strain Lactobacillus rhamnosus GG (LGG) in ADHD: Children and Adolescents Report Better Health-Related Quality of Life. *Front. Psychiatry* **2020**, *11*, 181. [CrossRef] [PubMed]
47. Liu, Y.-W.; Liong, M.T.; Chung, Y.-C.E.; Huang, H.-Y.; Peng, W.-S.; Cheng, Y.-F.; Lin, Y.-S.; Wu, Y.-Y.; Tsai, Y.-C. Effects of Lactobacillus Plantarum PS128 on Children with Autism Spectrum Disorder in Taiwan: A Randomized, Double-Blind, Placebo-Controlled Trial. *Nutrients* **2019**, *11*, 820. [CrossRef] [PubMed]
48. Dieterich, W.; Tietz, E.; Kohl, M.; Konturek, P.C.; Rath, T.; Neurath, M.F.; Zopf, Y. Food Intolerance of Unknown Origin: Caused by Mucosal Inflammation? A Pilot Study. *Clin. Transl. Gastroenterol.* **2021**, *12*, e00312. [CrossRef]

49. Farin, H.F.; Karthaus, W.R.; Kujala, P.; Rakhshandehroo, M.; Schwank, G.; Vries, R.G.; Kalkhoven, E.; Nieuwenhuis, E.E.; Clevers, H. Paneth Cell Extrusion and Release of Antimicrobial Products is Directly Controlled by Immune Cell–Derived IFN-γ. *J. Exp. Med.* **2014**, *211*, 1393–1405. [CrossRef] [PubMed]
50. Stevenson, J.; Buitelaar, J.; Cortese, S.; Ferrin, M.; Konofal, Éric; Lecendreux, M.; Simonoff, E.; Wong, I.C.K.; Sonuga-Barke, E.; The European ADHD Guidelines Group. Research Review: The Role of Diet in the Treatment of Attention-Deficit/Hyperactivity Disorder-An Appraisal of the Evidence on Efficacy and Recommendations on the Design of Future Studies. *J. Child. Psychol. Psychiatry* **2014**, *55*, 416–427. [CrossRef] [PubMed]

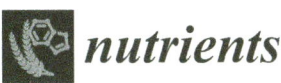

Review

Effects of Caffeine Consumption on Attention Deficit Hyperactivity Disorder (ADHD) Treatment: A Systematic Review of Animal Studies

Javier C. Vázquez [1,2,*], Ona Martin de la Torre [1,2], Júdit López Palomé [3] and Diego Redolar-Ripoll [1,2]

[1] Faculty of Psychology and Educational Sciences, Cognitive NeuroLab, Universitat Oberta de Catalunya, 08018 Barcelona, Spain; odominguezma@uoc.edu (O.M.d.l.T.); dredolar@uoc.edu (D.R.-R.)
[2] Neuromodulation Unit, Institut Brain 360, 08022 Barcelona, Spain
[3] Consorci d'Educació de Barcelona, Centre de Màxima Complexitat Elisenda de Montcada, Generalitat de Catalunya, 08010 Barcelona, Spain; jlope284@xtec.cat
* Correspondence: jcorreav@uoc.edu

Citation: Vázquez, J.C.; Martin de la Torre, O.; López Palomé, J.; Redolar-Ripoll, D. Effects of Caffeine Consumption on Attention Deficit Hyperactivity Disorder (ADHD) Treatment: A Systematic Review of Animal Studies. *Nutrients* 2022, *14*, 739. https://doi.org/10.3390/nu14040739

Academic Editors: Edward D. Barker and Marilyn Cornelis

Received: 23 December 2021
Accepted: 8 February 2022
Published: 10 February 2022

Publisher's Note: MDPI stays neutral with regard to jurisdictional claims in published maps and institutional affiliations.

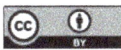

Copyright: © 2022 by the authors. Licensee MDPI, Basel, Switzerland. This article is an open access article distributed under the terms and conditions of the Creative Commons Attribution (CC BY) license (https://creativecommons.org/licenses/by/4.0/).

Abstract: Attention deficit hyperactivity disorder (ADHD) is a neurodevelopmental disorder characterized by a persistent pattern of inattention and/or hyperactivity-impulsivity. ADHD impairments arise from irregularities primarily in dopamine (DA) and norepinephrine (NE) circuits within the prefrontal cortex. Due to ADHD medication's controversial side effects and high rates of diagnosis, alternative/complementary pharmacological therapeutic approaches for ADHD are needed. Although the number of publications that study the potential effects of caffeine consumption on ADHD treatment have been accumulating over the last years, and caffeine has recently been used in ADHD research in the context of animal models, an updated evidence-based systematic review on the effects of caffeine on ADHD-like symptoms in animal studies is lacking. To provide insight and value at the preclinical level, a systematic review based on PRISMA guidelines was performed for all publications available up to 1 September 2021. Caffeine treatment increases attention and improves learning, memory, and olfactory discrimination without altering blood pressure and body weight. These results are supported at the neuronal/molecular level. Nonetheless, the role of caffeine in modulating ADHD-like symptoms of hyperactivity and impulsivity is contradictory, raising discrepancies that require further clarification. Our results strengthen the hypothesis that the cognitive effects of caffeine found in animal models could be translated to human ADHD, particularly during adolescence.

Keywords: caffeine; attention deficit hyperactivity disorder; impulsivity; ADHD; animal models

1. Introduction

Attention Deficit Hyperactivity Disorder (ADHD) is the most commonly diagnosed and treated mental disorder during childhood [1] and it is increasingly diagnosed and treated in during adulthood [2]. ADHD is a neurodevelopmental disorder characterized by a pattern of inattention and/or hyperactivity-impulsivity, persisting no less than six months, that is inconsistent with developmental level and has negative impact in at least two settings (academic, occupational or social) [3]. Inattention refers to important difficulties in sustaining attention to tasks that do not deliver a high level of stimulation or regular rewards, distractibility, and difficulties with organisation. Hyperactivity refers to disproportionate motor activity and difficulties with remaining still, most manifest in structured situations that involve behavioral self-control. Finally, impulsivity is a propensity to behave in response to immediate stimuli, without consideration of the risks and consequences [4]. Specific manifestations vary across individuals, and may change over the course of development. Depending on the symptoms presented, three different types of ADHD can be diagnosed: predominantly inattentive presentation, predominantly hyperactive-impulsive presentation, or combined presentation [3,4]. Although ADHD onset occurs during childhood and it often persists into adulthood, there is an important knowledge gap concerning

ADHD lifespan aspects [5]. Population surveys suggest that ADHD occurs in most cultures in about 5% of children and about 2.5% of adults [6] and, as of 2019, it was estimated to affect 84.7 million people worldwide [7]. ADHD management recommendations depend on the country [8–10] and usually include psychotherapy (essentially Cognitive Behavior Therapy, CBT), lifestyle changes and medications [11]. ADHD medication treatment, however, has been historically considered controversial [12], particularly due to its side effects [13–15]. In the face of these controversies and high rates of diagnosis, alternative/complementary pharmacological therapeutic approaches for ADHD are needed.

Although larger ADHD models containing supplementary pathways have been suggested [16,17], it is widely accepted that ADHD impairments, including selective and sustained attention, impulsivity, and motor activity, arise from abnormalities in different circuits involving the prefrontal cortex [18]: sustained attention is modulated by a cortico-striato-thalamocortical (CSTC) loop that comprises the dorsolateral prefrontal cortex (DLPFC) projecting to the striatal complex. Selective attention is modulated by a cortico-striato-thalamo-cortical (CSTC) loop ascending from the dorsal anterior cingulate cortex (dACC) and projecting to the striatal complex, followed by the thalamus, and back to the dACC. Impulsivity is related to a cortico-striato-thalamocortical (CSTC) loop that contains the orbitofrontal cortex (OFC), the striatal complex, and the thalamus. Finally, motor activity, including hyperactivity and psychomotor agitation or retardation, can be modulated by a cortico-striato-thalamo-cortical (CSTC) loop arising from the prefrontal motor cortex to the lateral striatum to the thalamus and back to the prefrontal motor cortex. ADHD patients cannot activate prefrontal cortex areas in an appropriate manner when responding to cognitive tasks requiring attention and executive control, and show a dysfunction in reward and motivation, hindering cognitive control of behaviour [19,20]. Children diagnosed with ADHD, in this regard, need stronger incentives to adapt their behaviour [21], showing impaired responses to partial schedules of reinforcement and difficulties in delaying gratification [22,23].

In ADHD, inefficient information processing and arousal-related behaviours are hypothetically caused by imbalances mainly in the dopamine (DA) and norepinephrine (NE) circuits [24,25] and the serotonin (5-HT), glutamate (GLU), and acetylcholine (ACh) pathways within these areas of the brain [26–28].

Different genes are associated with the disorder, including the serotonin transporter (SERT), the synaptosomal-associated protein (SNAP-25), and the brain-derived neurotrophic factor (BDNF) [29,30], while some genes directly affect DA neurotransmission, including the DA transporter (DAT) or the DA receptor 4 (DRD4) [31,32]. In this respect, the ventral tegmental area (VTA) and locus coeruleus (LC) neurons have different targets, although their efferent fibers converge into the PFC: DA is released into the nucleus accumbens (NAcc), facilitating reward; NE is released in different posterior cortical areas, optimizing the organism reaction to significant stimuli; and both organic compounds are released into the PFC, enhancing working memory and attention in the face of significant stimuli [33].

Animal studies have provided insights into the pathological and neurochemical basis of ADHD through different types of animal model (see Figure 1) [34]. Among these, the spontaneously hypertensive rat (SHR) is considered an excellent and validated hyperactive model to study ADHD. Concerning its behavioral profile, SHR presents anomalies in DA neurotransmission [35] and, importantly, in adenosine neurotransmission [36].

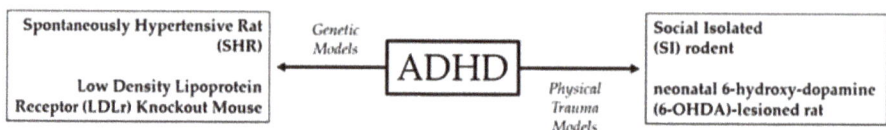

Figure 1. Animal models of Attention Deficit Hyperactivity Disorder. Key for abbreviations used: SHR: spontaneously hypertensive rat, low-density lipoprotein receptor, SI: social isolated, 6-OHDA: 6-hydroxy-dopamine, ADHD: Attention Deficit Hyperactivity Disorder.

Caffeine, in this respect, is an adenosine A_1 and A_{2A} receptor antagonist controlling synaptic plasticity [37]. These receptors are functionally paired with certain postsynaptic DA receptors, such as D2 receptors, where DA binds and has a stimulatory effect. When adenosine binds to its receptors, this causes reduced sensitivity of D2 receptors. Antagonism of adenosine receptors by caffeine prevents adenosine from binding, enhancing dopaminergic actions [18,24]. In addition to these dopaminergic effects, it has been shown that caffeine also produces secondary effects on ACh and NE [37–39]. Moreover, caffeine's effects on the non-selective antagonism of adenosine receptors also generate vasoconstriction in the nervous system. In this respect, it has been shown that caffeine modifies the blood perfusion signal, measured by fMRI, due to its neural and vascular effects, depending on the cerebral distribution of its receptors [40]. Similarly, the effect that caffeine may have at the cognitive level could depend on its regional effects on vascular response [41].

Nevertheless, the potential of caffeine consumption as a treatment for ADHD remains largely controversial, with studies showing efficacy in relieving ADHD-related symptoms [42], and studies failing to find superior effects when compared to first-line ADHD medication [43]. Beyond ADHD, there is an existing correlation between the daily consumption of moderate doses of caffeine and related benefits in different psychiatric disorders linked with adenosine A_{2A} receptor blockade controlling synaptic plasticity [44], mainly at the glutamatergic synapses [45]. Moreover, regular coffee consumption improves children's performance in comparison to decaffeinated coffee or placebo [46]. However, some studies have reported that caffeine consumption improvement is not significantly superior to placebo [47] or methylphenidate (MPD) [48], while hyperactivity has been strongly associated with higher coffee consumption among adolescents [49].

The number of publications that study the potential effects of caffeine consumption on ADHD treatment has accumulated since 1975 (see Figure 2) and, over the last few years, caffeine has been used in ADHD research in the context of animal models. Surprisingly, an updated evidence-based systematic review on the effects of caffeine on ADHD-like symptoms in animal studies is lacking.

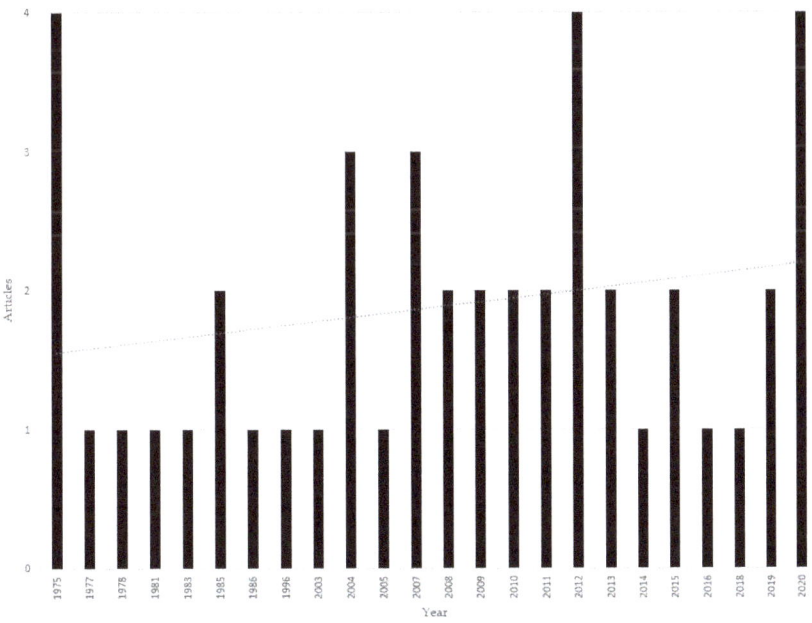

Figure 2. Caffeine/Attention Deficit Hyperactivity Disorder-related articles since 1975 (Source: MEDLINE).

Consequently, to provide insight and value at the preclinical level, we sought to produce a comprehensive compilation and systematically review all the relevant scientific publications that make reference to the underlying effects of caffeine intake on treating ADHD-like symptoms in animal studies.

2. Materials and Methods

We conducted a systematic review of ADHD research in the context of animal models to assess the association between caffeine and ADHD-dependent variables including attention, locomotor activity, impulsive behavior, learning, and memory.

2.1. Search Strategy

Figure 3 depicts the search strategy. We followed the guidelines and recommendations contained in the Preferred Reporting Items for Systematic Reviews and Meta-Analyses (PRISMA) statement [50], in order to reliably structure the gathered information in this systematic review. Academic articles were located using two electronic databases: MEDLINE and Web of Science. Only the results from these two databases were reported, since results from other sources (Scopus, Google Scholar) did not provide any relevant new results. No restrictions regarding publication date were applied. The literature search was conducted on 5 September 2021.

According to our proposal, the MEDLINE search strategy was established on the following key search terms: "caffeine" [Mesh] AND "Attention Deficit Disorder with Hyperactivity" [Mesh]. MeSH (Medical Subject Headings) terms were therefore used in the development of this search. The Web of Science search strategy was based on the following key search terms: ("attention" OR "hyperactivity" OR "ADHD") AND "caffeine".

2.2. Study Selection Criteria

The search was limited to preclinical and original experiments on non-human animals. The inclusion criteria were: (1) English-written, indexed studies; (2) non-human animal preclinical/experimental studies; (3) the mention of the relationship between caffeine treatment and ADHD-like symptoms; and (4) controlled studies with separately treated groups. The exclusion criteria were: (1) clinical/experimental/qualitative studies on humans; (2) not mentioning caffeine treatment and ADHD-like symptoms at all; (3) reviews, posters, conference abstracts, oral speeches, commentaries, theoretical papers, unpublished relevant studies, and other studies relevant to the topic but not published in peer-reviewed journals; and (4) case and cross-over studies.

2.3. Study Selection

Duplicates of all the databases were removed. Titles and abstracts were independently screened by two authors (J.C.V. and O.M.d.l.T.) according to the inclusion and exclusion criteria. Articles interpreted as compatible were selected for a full-text analysis to determine whether they were or were not within the inclusion criteria. Furthermore, the references of selected studies were screened in search of additional articles that met the inclusion criteria. Whenever a divergence of opinions emerged, a third author (D.R.-R.) was consulted to discuss and reach an agreement between the authors.

2.4. Data Extraction and Analyses

Following selection of the studies, data were extracted and prearranged into a table. The subsequent information was collected: (1) author/s and year; (2) species: strain, sex, and sample (n); (3) animal model; (4) age; (5) independent variables; (6) caffeine treatment; (7) behavioral tests/types of stress; (8) dependent variables; and (9) main results.

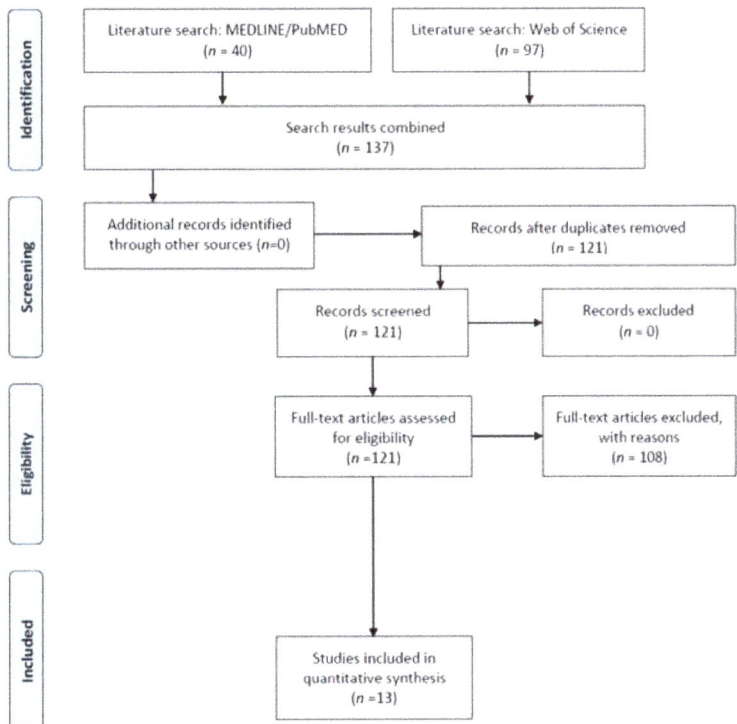

Figure 3. Flow diagram of study's selection based on PRISMA guidelines [50].

3. Results

Due to the large number of results acquired by the search terms, strict inclusion/exclusion criteria were applied to limit the final selection of studies. Figure 2 shows the studies included in quantitative synthesis.

3.1. Study Selection

A total of 121 unique citations was initially retrieved through the combined search, after which 108 citations were excluded after full-text screening because they did not meet the inclusion criteria. Therefore, 13 studies (Pandolfo et al., 2013 [51]; Ouichi et al., 2013 [52]; Caballero et al., 2011 [53]; Ruiz-Oliveira et al., 2019 [54]; Higgins et al., 2007 [55]; França et al., 2020 [56]; Nunes et al., 2018 [57]; Szczepanik et al., 2016 [58]; Pires et al., 2010 [59]; Prediger et al., 2005 [60]; Leffa et al., 2019 [61]; Pires et al., 2009 [62]; Alves et al., 2020 [63]) on animal models were finally considered. Based on their methodology, the studies in this review could be classified as experimental ($n = 10$; 76.9%), randomly assigning the subjects sample to the experimental groups, and quasi-experimental ($n = 3$; 23.1%), where the groups were usually constructed according to the subject's characteristics. The first studies relevant to the topic were from 2005, while the most recent studies included in this review were published in 2020. Table 1 describes each article individually.

3.1.1. Species, Animal Model, Sex, and Treatment

Most of the animal studies were performed on rodents. Ten studies were conducted with rats and two with mice. Only one of the studies used zebrafish as an animal model. Four studies used only males, five used both males and females, and four used only females. Different caffeine treatments and routes of administration were used, along with different durations (Table 1). Chronic treatments were mainly performed by dilating caffeine powder in the system water, whereas acute treatments were mainly administered intraperitoneally (i.p.).

3.1.2. Animal Models of ADHD

Overall, nine studies used genetic animal models of ADHD: eight studies used SHR, and one study used the low-density lipoprotein receptor (LDLr) mouse. Finally, two studies used physical trauma to provide an epigenetic animal model of ADHD: one study caused 6-hydroxy-dopamine (6-OHDA) lesions in rats, while one study used social isolation (SI) as an intensely stressful environment in mice (Table 1).

3.1.3. Behavioral Tests

Five studies used the object recognition task; four studies used the Y maze test; three studies used the open field test; two studies used the water maze test; and two studies used the novel object recognition test. In addition, other tests were performed, including the water-finding test, the five-choice serial reaction time task (5-CSRTT), the locomotor activity test, the discrimination task, the Olton maze behavioral assay, the attention set-shifting task, the fear-conditioning test, the tolerance to delay of reward task, and the olfactory discrimination test. Finally, one study induced the animals to a certain type of stress by means of social isolation and aggressivity (Table 1).

3.2. Study Outcomes

The results are summarized in Table 1. Considering the amount of data provided in the reviewed articles, we decided to categorize all the information based on caffeine's effects on each relevant ADHD-like evaluated parameter, as follows.

3.2.1. Attention

Attention and Behavioral Flexibility

Pandolfo et al. [51] examined the impact of chronic caffeine treatment during adolescence on SHR and Wistar Kyoto (WKY) rats' performance in an attention set-shifting task, placing emphasis on response to conflict. The task was divided into different phases: familiarization, response discrimination, and visual cue discrimination. During the response discrimination phase, statistical analysis showed that vehicle-treated SHR needed a superior amount of trials to reach the benchmark of 10 consecutive correct choices, compared with WKY rats. Importantly, treatment with caffeine (2 mg/kg, i.p.) improved SHR discriminative learning in a selective manner, as indicated by a reduction in the number of trials needed to reach the benchmark, while treatment with caffeine had no effect on WKY rats. During the visual cue discrimination phase, SHR required more trials to master the task, compared with WKY rats. Once more, caffeine treatment (2 mg/kg, i.p.) diminished the number of trials needed to reach the benchmark. Finally, statistical analysis showed that vehicle-treated SHR made significantly more regressive and never-reinforced errors than vehicle-treated WKY rats. Remarkably, while treatment with caffeine (2 mg/kg, i.p.) diminished the number of these errors in SHR, it had no effect on WKY rats.

Table 1. Summary of included studies.

Author/s & Year	Species, Strain, Sex & Sample (n)	Animal Model	Age	Independent Variables	Caffeine Treatment	Behavioral Tests/ Type of Stress	Dependent Variables	Main Results
Szczepanik et al., 2016	Mice C57Bl/6 wild-type (8) LDLr (8) Female	Genetic (LDLr)	3 months 8 months	Treatment (caffeine or vehicle) Strain (C57Bl/6 wild type or LDLr)	10 mg/kg oral route Chronic treatment (21 days)	Open-field arena	Spontaneous locomotor activity (total distance travelled) Anxiety (time in the center) Exploratory behavior (visual inspection of the occupation plot)	- LDLr mice travelled greater distances than the C57Bl/6 wild type mice during the 5 min period of analysis. - Caffeine treatment induced a renormalization effect in 8 month-old mouse locomotion. - Caffeine treatment was unable to modify the hyperlocomotion observed in 3 month-old LDLr mice. - All animal groups spent a similar amount of time in the center of an open field. - Similar exploratory behavior between groups.
Higgins et al., 2007	Rats LE (15–16) CD (12–16) Male	Not used	Not specified	Treatment (caffeine, SCH412348, KW-6002, DPCPX, CGS-21680, amphetamine) Strain (LE or CD)	1 mL/kg i.p. route One dose, prior testing	Five-choice serial reaction time task Locomotor activity test	Selective attention (Correct/incorrect trials, omissions, premature and perseverative responses, choice accuracy, correct/incorrect, and magazine latency) Hypolocomotion (distance travelled)	- Caffeine, SCH 412348 and KW-6002 augmented time reaction in LE and CD, without effect on accuracy. - Effects of SCH 412348 were at doses that were not overtly psychostimulatory. - CGS-21680 reduced speed reaction and augmented omissions. A CGS-21680 lower dose reduced the increased premature response caused by amphetamine. - Caffeine's attentional-enhancing effects were facilitated through A_{2A} receptor blockade. Selective A_{2A} receptor antagonists could be included as a potential therapy for ADHD.
Ruiz-Oliveira et al., 2019	Zebrafish wild-type (40) Male Female	Not used	4 months	Treatment (caffeine or vehicle)	10 mg/L 50 mg/L drinking water Chronic treatment (14 days)	Discrimination task	Conditioned learning ability (average swimming speed, intergroup freezing, maximum speed, time spent in each area, latency to enter each area)	- 0 and 10 mg/L caffeine groups spent most of the time close to the target. - 10 mg caffeine group had the shortest latency to reach the target. - 0 and 10 mg/L caffeine groups increased the average speed and distance travelled. - Caffeine exposure at low doses seems to enhance visual cue discrimination and zebrafish performance.
Prediger et al., 2005	Rats WKY (7–8) SHR (7–8) Female	Genetic (SHR)	3 months	Treatment (caffeine or vehicle) Strain (WKY or SHR)	1.3 mg/kg 10 mg/kg i.p. route One dose, prior testing	Water maze task	Spatial learning (escape latency, distance travelled, swimming speed) Mean arterial pressure	- SHR needed a larger amount of trials during the training session to learn the spatial information, although a similar profile to that of WKY rats during the test session, showing a selective spatial learning deficit. - Caffeine's pre-training administration enhanced SHRs' spatial learning deficit. - Caffeine's post-training administration did not enhance SHRs' test performance, although it improved WKY rats' memory retention. - Mean blood pressure was not altered by caffeine.

Table 1. Cont.

Author/s & Year	Species, Strain, Sex & Sample (n)	Animal Model	Age	Independent Variables	Caffeine Treatment	Behavioral Tests/ Type of Stress	Dependent Variables	Main Results
Pires et al., 2009	Rats WKY (15) SHR (18) Male Female	Genetic (SHR)	3 months	Treatment (MPD, DPCPX, caffeine, ZM241385 or vehicle) Strain (WKY or SHR)	1 mg/kg 3 mg/kg 10 mg/kg i.p. route One dose, prior testing	Object recognition task	Object recognition (investigation time, discrimination time) Mean arterial pressure	- SHR only discriminated between the most structurally distinct pairs of objects. - Pre-training administration of MPD, caffeine, the selective adenosine receptor antagonists DPCPX and ZM241385, or the association of ineffective doses of DPCPX and ZM241385, improved the performance of SHR in the object-recognition task. - The administration of the same doses of MPD and caffeine did not significantly alter the mean arterial pressure of either WKYs or SHRs.
Pires et al., 2010	Rats WKY (37) SHR (38) Female	Genetic (SHR)	25/38 days	Treatment (caffeine, MPD or vehicle) Strain (WKY or SHR)	3 mg/kg i.p. Route. Chronic treatment (14 days)	Object recognition task	Object recognition (investigation time, discrimination time) Spontaneous locomotor activity Mean arterial pressure Body weight	- WKY rats distinguished all the items. SHRs were unable to distinguish pairs of items with slight structural alterations. - Caffeine or MPD chronic treatment enhanced SHR item-recognition deficits. The same treatments impaired the adult WKY rats' short-term object recognition ability. - Effects were independent of variations in locomotion, arterial blood pressure, and body weight.
Caballero et al., 2011	Rats 6-OHDA lesioned (9) Saline-lesioned (9) Male Female	Physical trauma (6-OHDA lesioned)	25 days	Treatment (caffeine or vehicle)	1 mg/mL drinking water Chronic treatment (14 days)	Olton maze behavioral assay	Motor behavior (number of arms crossed) Attention behavior (total number of arms walked, and total number of arms walked until one was repeated)	- Caffeine treatment significantly improved 6-OHDA lesioned rats' attention deficit. - After caffeine consumption, no changes were found in motor activity.

Table 1. Cont.

Author/s & Year	Species, Strain, Sex & Sample (n)	Animal Model	Age	Independent Variables	Caffeine Treatment	Behavioral Tests/ Type of Stress	Dependent Variables	Main Results
Pandolfo et al., 2013	Rats WKY (16) SHR (16) Male	Genetic (SHR)	24 days	Treatment (caffeine or vehicle (saline)) Strain (WKY or SHR)	2 mg/kg i.p. route Chronic treatment (twice daily for 21 days)	Attentional-set shifting; anxiety-related behavior; Y maze; locomotion-related behavior	Attention (regressive and never-reinforced errors, perseverative errors, total number of trials required before reaching 10 correct consecutive choices); Locomotion and anxiety (number of peripheral squares crossed, number of central squares crossed, percentage of central locomotion) Spatial recognition (number of entries; time spent per arm; random exploration)	- SHRs were hyperactive and showed poorer performance in the attentional set-shifting and Y-maze paradigms, displayed increased dopamine transporter density, and increased dopamine uptake in frontocortical and striatal terminals. - Chronic caffeine treatment improved memory and attention deficits, and normalized dopaminergic function in SHR. - First indication of adenosine A_{2A} receptors ($A_{2A}R$) in nerve terminals in frontal cortex. - First evidence that $A_{2A}R$ density is improved in SHR.
Ouichi et al., 2013	Mice ICR (9) Male Female	Physical trauma (SI)	4 weeks	Treatment (MPD and caffeine) SI	0.5–1 mg/kg i.p. route One dose, prior testing	Water-finding test; aggression; modified Y-maze test; novel object recognition test; fear-conditioning test	Spatial attention (entering & drinking latency) Aggression (duration of wrestling) Spatial recognition (time spent in the new arm; total time exploring objects) Fear conditioning (freezing behavior)	- SI rats showed deficits in spatial attention on the water-finding test. Re-socialized did not reduce deficit in spatial attention. SI effect on spatial attention revealed no difference in gender or correlation with aggressive behaviour. - SI impaired conditional and contextual fear memory. - MPD and caffeine enhanced deficits in SI-induced latent learning in a manner that was reversible with cholinergic but not dopaminergic antagonists.

Table 1. Cont.

Author/s & Year	Species, Strain, Sex & Sample (n)	Animal Model	Age	Independent Variables	Caffeine Treatment	Behavioral Tests/ Type of Stress	Dependent Variables	Main Results
Nunes et al., 2018	Rats WKY (5–15) SHR (5–15) Male Female	Genetic (SHR)	15 days 28 days 50 days	Treatment (caffeine/water) Strain (WKY or SHR)	caffeine/caffeine or water 0.3 g/L drinking water Until PND 28	Open-field test; Novel object recognition; Y maze task	Open field test (travel distance periphery) Habituation (total travelled distance in the open field) Spatial recognition- Y maze and object recognition (exploration, discrimination ratio, number of entries, time spent in novel arm, total number of entries in three arms)	- Adolescent SHR from both sexes displayed hyperlocomotion, recognition, and spatial memory disturbances. Females displayed a lack of habituation and deteriorated spatial memory. - Caffeine was effective at improving recognition memory damage in both sexes. - Spatial memory was improved only in female SHRs. - Female SHRs displayed impaired hyperlocomotion following caffeine treatment. - SHRs of both sexes presented increases in BDNF, truncated and phospho-TrkB receptors, and phospho-CREB levels in the hippocampus. - Caffeine normalized BDNF in males and truncated TrkB receptor in both sexes.
Leffa et al., 2019	Rats WKY (7–9) SHR (7–9) Male	Genetic (SHR)	60/65 days 24 days	Treatment (WIN, AM251, caffeine or vehicle) Strain (WKY or SHR)	2 or 5 mg/kg i.p. route Acute pretreatment, one dose Chronic treatment (21 days)	Tolerance to delay of reward; T maze	Impulsive behavior (tolerance to delay of reward)	- WIN treatment decreased large reward choices and AM251 treatment increased large reward choices in SHR. - Acute caffeine pretreatment blocked WIN effects. - Chronic caffeine treatment increased the impulsive phenotype and potentiated the WIN effects. - Cannabinoid and adenosine receptors modulate impulsive behavior in SHR.
Alves et al., 2020	Rats-pregnant SHR (40–70) WKY (40–70) Female	Genetic (SHR)	In vitro	Treatment (caffeine, DMSO, LY294002, adenosine selective agonist and antagonists) Strain (WKY or SHR)	Caffeine incubation (30 µM) One dose	No behavioral task	Morphological alterations (singling, neurite branching)	- SHR neurons displayed less neurite branching, shorter maximal neurite length and decreased axonal outgrowth. - Caffeine recovered neurite branching and elongation from SHR neurons via PKA and PI3K signaling. - $A_{2A}R$ agonist (CGS 21680) promoted more neurite branching via PKA signaling. - The selective $A_{2A}R$ antagonist (SCH 58261) was efficient at recovering axonal outgrowth from SHR neurons through PI3K and not PKA signaling.

Table 1. Cont.

Author/s & Year	Species, Strain, Sex & Sample (n)	Animal Model	Age	Independent Variables	Caffeine Treatment	Behavioral Tests/ Type of Stress	Dependent Variables	Main Results
França et al., 2020	Rats WKY (9) SHR (11) Male	Genetic (SHR)	30 days 4–5 months	Treatment (caffeine or water) Physical exercise Strain (WKY or SHR)	0.3 mg/mL, drinking water One dose	Olfactory discrimination; Open field; Object recognition; Water maze	Olfactory discrimination (time spent in compartments, numbers of crossings) Locomotor activity (total distance, time spent in the central zone) Short-term memory (total time spent exploring the objects, discrimination index) Working and procedural memories (escape latency)	- SHR showed olfactory and short-term recognition memory deficiencies from adolescence to adulthood, accompanied by lower prefrontal cortex and hippocampus SNAP-25 levels. - Caffeine and physical exercise during adolescence or adulthood repaired the olfactory discrimination ability and enhanced short-term recognition memory in SHRs. - Caffeine consumption and physical exercise during adolescence augmented hippocampus and prefrontal cortex SNAP-25, syntaxin, and serotonin levels, as well as SHRs' striatal dopamine levels.

Key for abbreviations used: LDLr: low-density lipoprotein receptor, LE rat: Long-Evans rat, CD rat: Cesarean-derived rat, i.p.: intraperitoneally, WKY rat: wistar Kyoto rat, SHR: spontaneously hypertensive rat, MPD: methylphenidate, 6-OHDA: 6-hydroxy-dopamine, $A_{2A}R$: Adenosine A_{2A} receptors, ICR mice: Institute of Cancer Research mice, SI: social isolation, PND: postnatal day, BDNF: brain-derived neurotrophic factor, SNAP-25: synaptosomal-associated protein 25.

Spatial Attention

Ouchi et al. [52] tested the effect of SI on latent learning using the water-finding test, measuring entering latency and drinking latency. The authors eventually discussed the utility of SI as an ADHD epigenetic model. They socially isolated male or female Institute of Cancer Research (ICR) mice for one week or more. Subsequently, the animals displayed spatial attention deficit during the water-finding task. Five weeks of resocialization following one week of SI failed to improve this deficit. Drinking latency depended on how much attention the animal paid to environmental factors, including the location of a tap water nozzle, which they were exposed to in the training trial. Therefore, a decrease in drinking latency correlated with the animal remembering the position/location of the nozzle. Caffeine (0.3–1 mg/kg, i.p.) induced changes in drinking latency on the water-finding test, in this sense, significantly ameliorating SI-induced latent learning deficits in a dose-dependent manner, independently of gender or age.

Caballero et al. [53] examined caffeine's therapeutic use in neonatal 6-OHDA lesioned rats, which constitute another existing ADHD animal model. At postnatal day (PND) 7, the rats were lesioned at the left striatum with 6-OHDA. At PND 25, spatial attention was measured with an eight arm radial maze, the Olton maze. The animals were then placed in the maze. The total number of arms the animals walked before completing six out of eight, or until they repeated one of them, was measured. After 14 days of treatment with caffeine, administered ad libitum into the drinking water, the authors assessed caffeine's effects on the attention deficit of the animals, using the same task. Interestingly, the 6-OHDA lesioned rats significantly improved their attention deficit after caffeine treatment. Consequently, the authors highlighted the properties through which caffeine managed the attentional deficits occurring during the prepubertal period of ADHD.

Discrimination

Ruiz-Oliveira et al. [54] evaluated the effect of caffeine on zebrafish performance in a task requiring focus and attention, the discrimination task. The task took place in three phases: tank acclimation, training, and test. The authors used visual cues during the training trials and the test trials. Distractors, objects resembling the target, were used to confuse the fish and impair conditioning. The fish were exposed to different caffeine concentrations for 14 days: 0 mg/L (control), 10 mg/L (low), and 50 mg/L (high). Notably, low caffeine doses improved the fishes' ability to discriminate the cues and reach the target; the fish spent most of the time close to the target where the reward was offered, and showing the shortest latency to reaching the target. The higher dose impaired the fishes' ability to find the target; the fish demonstrated increased anxiety, a possible side effect of the substance.

Selective Attention

Higgins et al. [55] evaluated the effect of caffeine on Long–Evans (LE) and Cesarean-derived (CD) rat performance in a selective attention task, the 5-CSRTT. The effects of caffeine were compared to the selective A_{2A} antagonists, SCH 412348 and KW-6002, and the A_1 antagonist, DPCPX. Caffeine (3–10 mg/kg, i.p.) increased reaction time in both LE and CD rats, with no effect on accuracy, an effect replicated by SCH 412348 (0.1–1 mg/kg PO) and KW-6002 (1–3 mg/kg PO), but not DPCPX (3–30 mg/kg PO). The faster response speed was observed in both the CD and LE rat strains at 3 mg/kg, although increased premature responses were confined to the LE strain at the 10 mg/kg dose. These results suggest that the attention-enhancing effects of caffeine were mediated through A_{2A} receptor blockade. Selective A_{2A} receptor antagonists may therefore have potential as therapies for attention-related disorders, such as ADHD.

3.2.2. Hyperactivity and Impulsivity

Locomotor Activity

França et al. [56] tested the effect of caffeine on the hyperlocomotion characteristic of ADHD by examining locomotor activity. Caffeine consumption (0.3 mg/mL in drinking water) and physical exercise in running wheels for 6 weeks, either during adolescence (30 days old) or adulthood (4–5 months old), did not relate to changes in spontaneous locomotion in SHR, in an open field, during the 5 min habituation phase of the object recognition test. Ruiz-Oliveira et al. [54] studied the effects of caffeine on zebrafish (4 months old, wild type, both sexes). Low concentrations of caffeine (10 mg/L) affected locomotor parameters, increasing average speed and decreasing freezing behavior. Interestingly, the levels of freezing and locomotor behavior were the same for the 50 mg/L caffeine group and the control group. Nunes et al. [57] evaluated locomotor activity during the late childhood and the end of adolescence of male and female SHR, using an open field arena and measuring the total distance travelled in meters along the periphery during 5 min. Although caffeine (0.3 g/L) did not impact hyperlocomotion during late childhood (PND 28) in either sex, continuous treatment aggravated adolescent female SHR hyperactivity (PND 50), suggesting that the consumption of caffeine during childhood may aggravate hyperactivity in females, but only if the administration persists up to adolescence. Szczepanik et al. [58] demonstrated that young (3 months old) and middle-aged (8 months old) LDLr mice display different responses to chronic caffeine treatment in terms of motor activity. Although caffeine was unable to modify the hyperlocomotion observed in 3 months old LDLr mice, caffeine attenuated the increased locomotor activity observed in 8 months old LDLr mice. Pandolfo et al. [51] tested whether chronic treatment with caffeine was able to counteract the hyperlocomotion characteristic of ADHD in SH, during the open field test. Chronic treatment with caffeine did not alter central and total locomotion in SHR. Similarly, Pires et al. [59] showed that chronic treatment with caffeine did not produce changes in SHR locomotion during the object recognition task sample phase. Interestingly, Caballero et al. [53] showed that neonatal 6-OHDA lesioned rats, a different ADHD animal model, demonstrated a non-significant tendency to decrease their motor activity after ad libitum caffeine consumption throughout the prepubertal period during an Olton maze behavioral assay. Higgins et al. [55] conducted two separate types of locomotor activity study. In a CGS-21680-induced hypolocomotion assay, pretreatment with caffeine (3–30 mg/kg, i.p.) produced a significant attenuation of the CGS-21680 hypolocomotion at different doses, of 10 mg/kg and 30 mg/kg, in CD rats. In a second experiment, caffeine (1–30 mg/kg, i.p.) produced a dose-related increase in locomotion in the animals habituated to the test chambers. Finally, Prediger et al. [60] did not find a direct increase in locomotor performance in SHR after the administration of acute doses of caffeine (1–10 mg/kg i.p.) when using a spatial version of the Morris water maze. No alteration was observed in the swimming speed in this regard.

Impulsive Behavior

Leffa et al. [61] focused on impulsive behavior to clarify the neurobiology of ADHD. They treated SHRs with caffeine, a non-selective adenosine receptor antagonist, to assess the modulating effects of the adenosine systems on tolerance to the delay of a reward. The animals had to choose between a small, but immediate, or a large, but delayed, reward. An acute pretreatment with caffeine (2 mg/kg or 5 mg/kg) increased number of large-reward choices. Conversely, chronic treatment with caffeine (2 mg/kg, for 21 days) augmented the impulsive phenotype and decreased the number of large-reward choices.

3.2.3. Learning and Memory

Non-Associative Learning

Habituation is a form of non-associative learning in which the animal's innate response to a stimulus decreases after prolonged or repeated presentations of this stimulus. Nunes et al. [57] analyzed habituation during late childhood and the end of adolescence in male and female SHRs. The authors observed a sex and age difference in habituation, with female SHRs showing lack of habituation from childhood onwards, and male SHRs showing a lack of habituation in adolescence. These difficulties observed in female habituation, however, were overturned by treatment with caffeine (0.3 g/L) during childhood.

Working Memory

The object recognition task is recognized as a working-memory task, relies on the animal's natural tendency for novelty, and tests the ability to discriminate between familiar and unfamiliar objects. França et al. [56] assessed working memory using an adapted version of the object recognition task, conducted in an open field during three different phases: habituation, sample and discrimination. Although the study results indicated that the disruption of the short-term recognition memory persisted into adulthood, the association of caffeine (0.3 mg/mL) and exercise during adulthood and adolescence improved short-term recognition memory in the SHR strain. Nunes et al. [57] also carried out the novel object recognition test and observed similar recognition memory disturbances in adolescent SHRs of both sexes. Nonetheless, caffeine intake (0.3 g/L) restricted to childhood restored recognition memory in adolescent SHRs of both sexes. To evaluate the potential of caffeine in ADHD therapy, Pires et al. [59] treated female WKY rats and SHR with caffeine (3 mg/kg, i.p.) for 14 consecutive days during the prepubertal period. The animals were tested during the object recognition test in the course of adulthood. While WKY rats discriminated between all the used objects, the SHRs were unable to differentiate between pairs of objects with subtle structural differences. Nonetheless, caffeine or MPD chronic treatment improved the deficits in object recognition in SHR. Pires et al. [62] showed, for the first time, the significant impairment of SHRs' short-term object-recognition ability in comparison with WKY rats. They further investigated the effects of caffeine (1, 3 or 10 mg/kg), 30 min before the sample phase, on the performance of WKY rats and SHR of both sexes in the object recognition task. The injection of caffeine (1, 3 or 10 mg/kg, i.p.) improved the discrimination index of female SHRs, while the highest tested dose of caffeine (10 mg/kg, i.p.) increased the discrimination index of male SHRs.

Spatial Learning

The water maze task is a behavioral procedure widely used with rodents to study spatial learning or spatial memory. Prediger et al. [60] used a circular swimming pool to assess the effect of caffeine administration on spatial learning deficit in SHRs. Adult female WKY rats and SHRs were treated with caffeine (1–10 mg/kg i.p.) before or immediately after training, or before the test session. Spatial learning deficit in SHR was improved through the pre-training administration of caffeine (1–10 mg/kg i.p.). SHR test performance was not altered by the post-training administration of caffeine (3 mg/kg i.p.), although WKY rats' memory retention was increased. Although França et al. [25] observed procedural memory impairment in adolescent SHRs during a cued version of the water maze, these normalized in adulthood.

Spatial Short-Term Memory

Given the willingness of rodents to explore new environments, the Y-Maze Test is widely used for testing the conditions affecting memory and learning. Pandolfo et al. [51] assessed SHRs' spatial short-term memory, using a Y-maze paradigm. When compared with WKY rats, the control group SHRs displayed a spatial learning deficit. Importantly, treatment with caffeine (2 mg/kg, i.p.) during adolescence improved SHR memory impairment. Nunes et al. [57] evaluated spatial memory in male and female SHRs using the Y-maze task at PND 53. Female SHRs showed worsened spatial memory. Although caffeine (0.3 g/L) showed effectiveness against recognition memory deficiency in males and females, only female SHRs increased the number of entries in the novel arm following caffeine treatment, from PND 15 to 55, and showed spatial memory recovery.

3.2.4. Olfactory Discrimination

França et al. [56] assessed the effects of caffeine consumption (0.3 mg/mL) and physical exercise on running on wheels over 6 weeks, during either adolescence (30 days old) or adulthood (4–5 months old), by means of SHR during the olfactory discrimination test. Besides providing the first evidence of deficits in olfactory discrimination in both adolescent and adult SHRs, the authors showed how caffeine, together with physical exercise, was able to restore olfactory discrimination ability in these animals during adolescence or adulthood.

3.2.5. Blood Pressure

França et al. [56] measured systolic blood pressure using the tail-cuff method in a non-invasive manner. For animals treated during adolescence, the systolic arterial pressure was measured before (basal values) and 14, 28, and 42 days after beginning the treatment, before the behavioral tests. For the rats subjected to caffeine treatment and physical exercise during adult life, two measurements were taken, one before the protocols (basal values) and the other after the last behavioral task. Notably, the hypertensive phenotype was not significantly altered by caffeine (0.3 mg/mL) or exercise. When applied from adolescence, caffeine and exercise had no effect on the development of hypertension and at 42 days of treatment (72 days of age), all the SHRs were hypertensive. For adult animals that were already hypertensive at the beginning of the treatment, no further significant differences between groups were observed. To investigate whether the SHRs' cognitive deficits could be directly associated with hypertension, Pires et al. [59] measured the effects of chronic caffeine administration (3 mg/kg, i.p.) during the prepubertal period on the arterial blood pressure of adult female WKY rats and female SHRs. The SHRs were hypertensive in comparison to the WKY control rats. The chronic administration of caffeine during the prepubertal period, at the same doses that reversed the cognitive deficits of adult SHR (3 mg/kg, i.p.), did not cause significant changes in blood pressure values in adulthood SHR and WKY rats. Again, Pires et al. [62] measured blood pressure after caffeine treatment to investigate whether the cognitive deficits of SHR could be directly related with hypertension. Accordingly, the arterial blood pressure (mmHg) of female WKY rats and female SHRs were measured 30 min after treatment with caffeine (1, 3, or 10 mg/kg, i.p.). As expected, the SHRs were hypertensive in comparison with the WKY control rats. However, the administration of the same doses of caffeine, which was able to improve the object discrimination deficits of the SHRs, did not significantly alter the mean arterial pressure of either the WKY rats or the SHRs. In a similar vein, Prediger et al. [60] measured the arterial blood pressure (mm Hg) of adult female WKY rats and SHRs 30 min after the injection of caffeine (1, 3 or 10 mg/kg, i.p.). Although the SHRs presented a significantly higher mean arterial pressure compared to the WKY control rats, treatment with caffeine did not significantly alter the mean arterial pressure of either the WKY or SHR groups. Caffeine was consequently able to improve the spatial learning deficits of the SHRs without varying their hypertensive state, showing that cognitive impairment in SHR might not be entirely explained by hypertension.

3.2.6. Body Weight

Pires et al. [59] measured the effects of chronic caffeine treatment during the prepubertal period on the body weight of juvenile and adult female WKY rats and female SHR. The body weights of the WKY rats and SHRs was were accordingly measured every 2 days during the treatment (14 days) with caffeine (1, 3, or 10 mg/kg, i.p.). The body weight of the adult rats also recorded during the performance of the object recognition task. Statistical comparisons indicated that juvenile rats from the SHR strain presented significantly lower mean body weight than the juvenile WKY rats. Notably, chronic treatment with caffeine did not alter the body weight of the evaluated rat strains. During adulthood, similar results for the body weight of the animals were found. Although significant strain differences were observed, chronic treatment with caffeine throughout the prepubertal period did not alter the final body weight of the animals in adulthood (regardless of strain). Likewise,

Pandolfo et al. (2013) [51] found no weight differences among groups following caffeine treatment (2 mg/kg, i.p.).

3.2.7. Neurobiology

Brain Levels of Synaptosomal-Associated Protein-25

França et al. [56] evaluated the effects of caffeine consumption (0.3 mg/mL in drinking water) and physical exercise on running wheels by measuring the brain levels of monoamine, using high-performance liquid chromatography, for 6 weeks. Regarding prefrontal cortex SNAP-25 levels, a statistical analysis revealed a significant increase in SNAP-25 levels in the prefrontal cortex in the group submitted to the combination of caffeine consumption with physical exercise. Regarding hippocampus SNAP-25 levels, the statistical analysis indicated a significant increase in hippocampal SNAP-25 levels selectively in animals submitted to the combination of caffeine consumption with physical exercise.

Brain Levels of Syntaxin

SNAP-25 is a component of the soluble N-ethylmaleimidesensitive factor attachment protein receptor (SNARE) complex, which is critical in regulating synaptic vesicle fusion and neurotransmitter release, along with syntaxin 1. Regarding prefrontal cortex syntaxin levels, a statistical analysis performed by França et al. (2020) [56] revealed a significant increase in syntaxin levels in the prefrontal cortex selectively in the group submitted to the combination of caffeine consumption and physical exercise. Regarding hippocampus syntaxin levels, the statistical analysis indicated a main effect of treatment with a marginal effect for treatment versus exercise interaction.

Brain Levels of Serotonin

França et al. [56] measured the effects of caffeine consumption and physical exercise throughout adolescence on serotonin (5-hydroxytryptamine, 5-HT) through high-performance liquid chromatography (HPLC). A statistical analysis performed by the authors showed that the combination of caffeine consumption and physical exercise during adolescence increased 5-HT levels in the prefrontal cortex of SHRs. Concerning hippocampal 5-HT levels, statistical comparisons showed that caffeine consumption and physical exercise, alone or in combination, significantly augmented hippocampal 5-HT levels.

Brain Levels of Dopamine

França et al. [56] evaluated dopamine levels in the prefrontal cortex, hippocampus, and striatum by using HPLC. Dopamine levels were not detectable in the hippocampus. Although a significant effect of treatment was observed in the prefrontal cortex, no significant effects were observed for exercise or their interaction. Statistical comparisons indicated no significant differences between groups in the levels of dopamine in the prefrontal cortex. Notably, the statistical analysis revealed significant effects of treatment, exercise, and their interaction on striatal dopamine levels. Subsequent statistical comparisons showed that caffeine intake and physical exercise, alone or in combination, significantly augmented striatal dopamine levels.

Dopamine Transporter Density

Pandolfo et al. [51] examined if the cognitive and attentional deficits of SHR and their attenuation by caffeine treatment were associated with alterations in the density of DAT in frontocortical and striatal terminals. The number of animals analyzed was four in the WKY control group, four in the WKY caffeine-treated group, three in the SHR control group, and four in the SHR caffeine-treated group. Statistical analysis showed a significant effect of the interaction between strain and treatment in the density of DAT in striatal and frontocortical synaptosomes. Consequently, DAT density was increased in both SHR brain areas of SHR and, significantly, caffeine treatment (2 mg/kg) during adolescence attenuated this enhanced DAT density in both brain areas of the SHRs, while caffeine treatment had no effect on the WKY rats.

Dopamine Uptake

Pandolfo et al. [51] tested whether a higher frontocortical density of DAT in SHR was complemented by an augmented uptake of dopamine. The authors directly measured dopamine uptake by synaptosomes. The number of animals was four per group. Both frontocortical and striatal synaptosomes from the SHRs took up almost the double amount of (^{3}H) dopamine during the 3 min incubation period than the synaptosomes from the WYK rats. Remarkably, chronic treatment with caffeine (2 mg/kg, i.p.) significantly reduced the dopamine uptake by synaptosomes from both brain areas in the SHRs when compared to vehicle-treated SHRs, while caffeine had no effect on the WKY rats.

Adenosine A_{2A} Receptor Density

The effects of chronic caffeine intake are generally attributed to the antagonism of A_{2AR}. Consequently, Pandolfo et al. [51] compared the density of A_{2AR} in striatal and frontocortical terminals from SHR or WKY rats treated with caffeine or saline. The number of animals analyzed was four in the WKY control group, three in the WKY caffeine-treated group, four in the SHR control group, and four in the SHR caffeine-treated group. Statistical analysis indicated a significant effect of the interaction between strain and treatment on A_{2AR} density both in the striatum and in the frontal cortex. Notably, fronto-cortical nerve terminals in the SHRs displayed more colocalization between A_{2AR} and synaptophysin immunoreactivities than in the WKY rats. This provided the first direct demonstration of the presence of A_{2AR} in fronto-cortical nerve terminals, and the first indication that A_{2AR} density is improved in SHRs.

Colocalization of Dopamine Transporter and Adenosine A_{2A} Receptors

Chronic treatment with caffeine is proposed to operate through A_{2AR} and was shown to affect DAT density and function. Pandolfo et al. [51] proved the colocalization of A_{2AR} and DAT in striatal and frontocortical nerve terminals. The number of animals analyzed was three in the WKY control group, four in the WKY caffeine-treated group, three in the SHR control group and three in the SHR caffeine-treated group. In the striatum, statistical analysis revealed a significant effect of strain on the colocalization of A_{2AR} and DAT immunoreactivities, and a subsequent comparison exhibited that nerve terminals from vehicle-treated SHR displayed a significantly lower colocalization of A_{2AR} and DAT in comparison with vehicle-treated WKY. In the frontal cortex, a statistical analysis revealed no significant effect of strain or treatment on the colocalization between A_{2AR} and DAT.

Brain-Derived Neurotrophic Factor

Nunes et al. [57] examined the effects of caffeine (0.3 g/L) administered from childhood onwards in the BDNF and its related proteins in both sexes of SHR rats. BDNF and its related proteins were therefore evaluated in the hippocampus of WKYs and SHRs of both sexes at PND 55. A statistical analysis revealed a significant effect of strain on BDNF levels, while the precursor form (proBDNF) remained unaltered. The TrkB receptor full length (TrkB-FL), phospho-TrkB, and truncated-form TrkB receptors were immunodetected in the hippocampuses of the WKYs and SHRs of both sexes. A statistical analysis revealed a significant effect of strain on the truncated form and also on phospho-TrkB. Furthermore, the transcription factor CREB was not altered either by strain or sex, although its phosphorylated form (phospho-CREB) was increased in the SHR hippocampus from both sexes. Finally, Nunes et al. [57] evaluated the impact of caffeine only on the BDNF levels and TrkB receptors (TrkB-FL, phospho-TrkB, and TrkB-T). Caffeine administered from PND 15 up to PND 55 (caff/caff) reduced the BDNF levels in the hippocampuses of SHR male rats, whereas the BDNF levels were unaltered in the SHR female rats in both schedules of treatment. In the male rats, caffeine in both schedules of treatment did not change either

TrkB-FL or TrkB-T levels, whereas female SHRs showed reduced TrkB-FL and TrkB-T forms as a consequence of caffeine treatment. Neither the increased phospho-TrkB nor the CREB were modified in the hippocampuses of the SHRs following caffeine treatment.

Neuronal Development In Vitro

Alves et al. [63] investigated caffeine's in vitro effects at the neuronal level. At first, SHR and WKY rats' cultured frontal cortical neurons were immunostained for MAP-2 during in vitro development. Later on, somatodendritic analyses were performed, measuring branch point number, root number, and maximal and total neurite length. Neurons from the SHRs displayed fewer differentiation patterns, including neurite branching, shorter maximal neurite length, and decreased axonal outgrowth. Following a 24 h period of caffeine incubation (30 µM), the SHR neurons showed an inferior percentage of zero branch points, and a superior percentage of two branch points. A trend toward a superior percentage of one-branch-point-neurons was observed for SHR neurons following treatment with caffeine. Caffeine also promoted a rise in the total and maximal neurite length in neurons from both strains. PKA or PI3K inhibitor were subsequently used to study whether one of the transducing systems activated by adenosine receptors, and in the neuronal differentiation, are responsible for the effects produced by caffeine. PKA inhibitor KT5720 (5 µM) did not change caffeine's ability to augment the percentage of SHR neurons with more branch points. Caffeine's effect on the recovery of the total neurite length of the SHR neurons was obstructed by PKA inhibitor. Comparable results were seen for maximal neurite length, in which PKA inhibitor completely decreased caffeine's effects. Finally, LY294002 (50 µM) was used as an inhibitor of PI3K and its presence blocked caffeine's effect on the increase in the number of branch points in SHR neurons. Furthermore, caffeine's effect on the prevention of reductions in the total neurite length were eliminated in the presence of PI3K inhibitor. Similar results were found for the maximal neurite length. The number of roots was also reduced by PI3K inhibitor in SHR neurons.

4. Discussion

ADHD is characterized by symptoms including attention deficits, impulsivity, and hyperactivity [3,4] that frequently persist throughout life [1,2,6]. Prefrontal cortex function modulation and attentional/behavioral regulation depends on the optimal release of signalling molecules such as NE, DA [24,25], as well as 5-HT, GLU, or ACh [26–28]. In this respect, genes, including the DAT or the DRD4 [31,32] or the SERT, the SNAP-25, and the BDNF [29,30], might play a role in causing ADHD. Therefore, agents that can lead to the optimal balance of these organic compounds are hypothetically beneficial in patients with ADHD by mainly returning prefrontal activity to adequate functional levels [18,33]. In this sense, it has long been discussed whether caffeine could become an effective pharmacological compound for the management of symptoms of ADHD [64,65].

This systematic review analyzed 13 animal studies that investigated the effects of caffeine on the modulation of ADHD-like symptoms. Overall, the reviewed results show that caffeine treatment increases attention and improves learning, memory, and olfactory discrimination without altering blood pressure and body weight.

Regarding attention, caffeine treatment improved the attentional and behavioral flexibility of SHRs [51], the spatial attention of 6-OHDA lesioned rats [53], and SI in ICR mice [52] during adolescence. Caffeine treatment improved the reaction time of LE and CD rats [55] and focus and attention in zebrafish [54] during adulthood.

Regarding learning and memory, caffeine treatment plus physical exercise during adulthood and adolescence improved working memory in SHRs [56]. In the same vein, caffeine treatment alone restored non-associative learning in female SHRs [57], improved working memory in SHRs [59], female SHRs [62], and adolescent SHRs [57]. The administration of caffeine improved spatial learning deficit in SHRs, increased memory retention in WKY rats [60], and improved spatial short-term memory in SHRs [51] and female SHRs [57].

Concerning olfactory discrimination, caffeine treatment, together with physical exercise, was able to restore olfactory discrimination in SHRs during adolescence or adulthood [56]. Concerning blood pressure, caffeine treatment did not alter the hypertensive phenotype in SHR [60,62] during adolescence or adult life [56], nor during the adult female SHR prepubertal period [59]. Finally, caffeine treatment did not alter body weight in SHRs [51,59].

If we are ever to acquire a truly in-depth understanding of ADHD pharmacotherapy, we need to face the following question: Does caffeine deserve a place in the battery of pharmacological agents for ADHD treatment, particularly during adolescence? Although previous meta-analyses [64] and reviews [65] were unable to provide any recommendations for adolescents diagnosed with ADHD, due to a lack of data, our reviewed results provide updated preclinical evidence and support the therapeutic potential of caffeine to improve attention, learning, memory, or olfactory discrimination in ADHD, especially during adolescence.

Beyond its clear effects on improving performance in tasks requiring attention, learning, memory and olfactory discrimination, without altering blood pressure and body weight, the implication of caffeine in modulating ADHD-like hyperactivity symptoms remains controversial. Indeed, caffeine treatment plus physical exercise did not affect locomotor activity in SHRs [56]. In a similar manner, caffeine treatment alone did not alter locomotion in SHR [51,59,60], preadolescent SHR [57], or young LDLr mice [58]. Nonetheless, caffeine treatment did increase locomotor activity in adolescent female SHRs [57], zebrafish [54]. Furthermore, it produced an increase related to dose in locomotion in CD rats and a significant attenuation of CGS-21680-induced hypolocomotion in CD rats [55], and it attenuated locomotor activity in middle-aged LDLr mice [58] and 6-OHDA lesioned rats throughout the prepubertal period [53]. This apparent discrepancy may have resulted from caffeine's promotion of different effects according to age and sex. In this regard, Nunes et al. [57] suggested that the intake of caffeine from the childhood period onwards may aggravate hyperactivity in females, if the consumption continues up to the adolescence period. Szczepanik et al. [58] linked the age-dependent effect induced by caffeine with the idea that the blockade of adenosine A_1/A_{2A} receptors attempts to renormalize a potentially maladaptive system [66], with age an important escalating factor in mice. In a different study, Ruiz-Oliveira et al. [54] proposed that caffeine-induced bursts of locomotion may be caused by a decrease in fatigue [67] rather than by an anxiogenic response. Importantly, the attenuation of motor activity by caffeine consumption was determined as a natural effect of growth rather than an effect of caffeine intake by Caballero et al. [53].

In terms of impulsivity, although acute pretreatment with caffeine increased the number of large reward choices made by SHRs, chronic treatment with caffeine increased the impulsive phenotype and decreased choices of large rewards by SHRs [61]. This discrepancy may be explained by previous studies performed on animal models of brain diseases, showing that while acute treatment acts mainly on A_1 receptors, chronic treatment acts mainly on A_{2A} receptors [68]. Leffa et al. [61], in this direction, underscored the ability of the adenosine modulation system to control behavioral inhibition.

Besides reviewing animal studies deciphering the effects of caffeine in the modulation of ADHD-like symptoms, we reviewed for the first time animal studies examining the effects of caffeine and adenosine receptors on neurons isolated from SHRs, at the neuronal level.

In this respect, treatment with caffeine and physical exercise during the adolescence period augmented the quantity of SNAP-25, syntaxin, and serotonin in the prefrontal cortex and the hippocampus, as well as striatal dopamine quantity, in SHRs [56]. In a similar manner, caffeine treatment alone during the adolescence period attenuated the improvement in DAT density in the fronto-cortical and striatal terminals of SHRs and diminished the dopamine uptake by synaptosomes from SHRs' fronto-cortical and striatal terminals [51]. Furthermore, Pandolfo et al. [51] demonstrated that fronto-cortical nerve terminals are provided with AdenosineA_{2A} receptor, the target of chronic caffeine exposure, whose density was found to be increased in SHRs. Caffeine treatment normalized BDNF levels in the hippocampuses of SHR males, while the same treatment normalized TrkB receptors TrkB-FL and TrkB-T SHR in the hippocampuses of SHR females [57]. Finally, neurons from SHRs showed an inferior number of zero-branch points, and a superior number of two-branch-points-neurons following in vitro caffeine treatment consisting of 24 h of caffeine incubation. After treatment with caffeine, an increase in the total and maximal neurite length and a tendency toward a superior number of one-branch-point neurons was also observed for SHR neurons. The effect of caffeine on increasing maximal neurite length, and on recuperating the entire neurite length of neurons from SHR, was entirely blocked by PKA inhibitor. LY294002, as an inhibitor of PI3K, blocked caffeine's effects on the increase in the amount of branch points in SHR neurons. Finally, the effect of caffeine on the prevention of reductions in the total neurite length, increasing maximal neurite length, and the number of roots was eradicated by the presence of PI3K inhibitor in SHR neurons [63].

5. Conclusions

Overall, our reviewed data suggest that caffeine is a possible adjuvant pharmacological strategy for the treatment of ADHD. The compiled preclinical data support the notion that caffeine improves ADHD-like symptoms of inattention and its related learning and memory impairments without affecting blood pressure and body weight. Our results are supported at the neuronal/molecular level, and strengthen the hypothesis that the cognitive effects of caffeine found in animal models of ADHD could be translated to humans diagnosed with the disorder, particularly during adolescence. Nonetheless, caution is needed when extrapolating potential effects identified in animal studies to human patients. In this work, studies that explored caffeine's effects on locomotor activity and impulsivity were contradictory, raising discrepancies that require further clarification. Although we consider that the reviewed results in this manuscript can potentially impact the scientific, pre-clinical, and clinical community and expand our knowledge regarding ADHD, more studies should be performed to validate our present knowledge while offering prospective clues to support caffeine as a therapeutic approach for the treatment of ADHD.

Author Contributions: J.C.V. contributed significantly to the conception and design of the manuscript, the acquisition of data, and data analysis and interpretation, agreeing to be responsible for all aspects of the work in ensuring that questions related to the accuracy or veracity of any part of the work are appropriately investigated and resolved. J.C.V., J.L.P., O.M.d.l.T. and D.R.-R. drafted the manuscript. D.R.-R. provided critical revision of the manuscript and final consent of the version to be published. All authors have read and agreed to the published version of the manuscript.

Funding: This research received no external funding.

Informed Consent Statement: Not applicable.

Data Availability Statement: Not applicable.

Acknowledgments: We thank William J. Giardino from Stanford University for helpful comments on this manuscript.

Conflicts of Interest: The authors declare no potential conflict of interest regarding the research, authorship, and/or publication of this article.

References

1. Ferguson, J.H. National Institutes of Health Consensus Development Conference Statement: Diagnosis and treatment of attention-deficit/hyperactivity disorder (ADHD). *J. Am. Acad. Child Adolesc. Psychiatry* **2000**, *39*, 182–193. [CrossRef] [PubMed]
2. Dopheide, J.A.; Pliszka, S.R. Attention-deficit-hyperactivity disorder: An update. *Pharmacotherapy* **2009**, *29*, 656–679. [CrossRef] [PubMed]
3. American Psychiatric Association. *Diagnostic and Statistical Manual of Mental Disorders: DSM-5*; American Psychiatric Association: Arlington, VA, USA, 2013.
4. ICD-11: 6A05 Attention Deficit Hyperactivity Disorder. Available online: https://icd.who.int/browse11/l-m/en#/http%3a%2f%2fid.who.int%2ficd%2fentity%2f821852937 (accessed on 22 December 2021).

5. Franke, B.; Michelini, G.; Asherson, P.; Banaschewski, T.; Bilbow, A.; Buitelaar, J.K.; Cormand, B.; Faraone, S.V.; Ginsberg, Y.; Haavik, J.; et al. Live fast, die young? A review on the developmental trajectories of ADHD across the lifespan. *Eur. Neuropsychopharmacol.* **2018**, *28*, 1059–1088. [CrossRef] [PubMed]
6. Tsuang, M.T.; Tohen, M.; Jones, P. *Textbook of Psychiatric Epidemiology*, 3rd ed.; John Wiley & Sons: Chichester, UK, 2011.
7. Global Health Metrics: Attention-Deficit/Hyperactivity Disorder—Level 3 Cause. Available online: https://www.thelancet.com/pb-assets/Lancet/gbd/summaries/diseases/adhd.pdf (accessed on 22 December 2021).
8. NICE Guideline [NG87]—Attention Deficit Hyperactivity Disorder: Diagnosis and Management. Available online: https://www.nice.org.uk/guidance/ng87/ (accessed on 22 December 2021).
9. Canadian ADHD Practice Guidelines. Available online: https://www.caddra.ca/cms4/pdfs/caddraGuidelines2011Introduction.pdf (accessed on 22 December 2021).
10. Centers for Disease Control and Prevention: ADHD Treatment Recommendations. Available online: https://www.cdc.gov/ncbddd/adhd/guidelines.html (accessed on 22 December 2021).
11. Wolraich, M.L.; Hagan, J.F.; Allan, C.; Chan, E.; Davison, D.; Earls, M.; Evans, S.W.; Flinn, S.K.; Froehlich, T.; Frost, J.; et al. Clinical practice guideline for the diagnosis, evaluation, and treatment of attention-deficit/hyperactivity disorder in children and adolescents. *Pediatrics* **2019**, *144*, e20192528. [CrossRef] [PubMed]
12. Schonwald, A.; Lechner, E. Attention deficit/hyperactivity disorder: Complexities and controversies. *Curr. Opin. Pediatr.* **2006**, *18*, 189–195. [CrossRef]
13. Wigal, S.B. Efficacy and safety limitations of attention-deficit hyperactivity disorder pharmacotherapy in children and adults. *CNS Drugs* **2009**, *23*, 21–31. [CrossRef]
14. Parker, J.; Wales, G.; Chalhoub, N.; Harpin, V. The long-term outcomes of interventions for the management of attention-deficit hyperactivity disorder in children and adolescents: A systematic review of randomized controlled trials. *Psychol. Res. Behav. Manag.* **2013**, *6*, 87. [CrossRef]
15. Arnold, L.E.; Hodgkins, P.; Caci, H.; Kahle, J.; Young, S. Effect of treatment modality on long-term outcomes in attention-deficit/hyperactivity disorder: A systematic review. *PLoS ONE* **2015**, *10*, e0116407. [CrossRef]
16. Castellanos, F.X.; Proal, E. Large-scale brain systems in ADHD: Beyond the prefrontal–striatal model. *Trends Cogn. Sci.* **2012**, *16*, 17–26. [CrossRef]
17. Cortese, S.; Kelly, C.; Chabernaud, C.; Proal, E.; Di Martino, A.; Milham, M.P.; Castellanos, F.X. Toward systems neuroscience of ADHD: A meta-analysis of 55 fMRI studies. *Am. J. Psychiatry* **2012**, *169*, 1038–1055. [CrossRef]
18. Stahl, S.M. *Stahl's Essential Psychopharmacology: Neuroscientific Basis and Practical Applications*, 4th ed.; Cambridge University Press: Cambridge, UK, 2013.
19. Haenlein, M.; Caul, W.F. Attention deficit disorder with hyperactivity: A specific hypothesis of reward dysfunction. *J. Am. Acad. Child Adolesc. Psychiatry* **1987**, *26*, 356–362. [CrossRef]
20. Johansen, E.B.; Killeen, P.R.; Russell, V.A.; Tripp, G.; Wickens, J.R.; Tannock, R. Origins of altered reinforcement effects in ADHD. *Behav. Brain Funct.* **2009**, *5*, 7. [CrossRef]
21. Kollins, S.H.; Lane, S.D.; Shapiro, S.K. The experimental analysis of childhood psychopathology: A matching analysis of the behavior of children diagnosed with Attention Deficit Hyperactivity Disorder. *Psychol. Record.* **1997**, *47*, 25–44. [CrossRef]
22. Sonuga-Barke, E.J. The dual pathway model of AD/HD: An elaboration of neuro-developmental characteristics. *Neurosci. Biobehav. Rev.* **2003**, *27*, 593–604. [CrossRef] [PubMed]
23. Tripp, G.; Wickens, J.R. Research review: Dopamine transfer deficit: A neurobiological theory of altered reinforcement mechanisms in ADHD. *J. Child Psychol. Psychiatry* **2008**, *49*, 691–704. [CrossRef]
24. Nestler, E.J.; Hyman, S.E.; Malenka, R.C.; Holtzman, D.M. *Molecular Neuropharmacology: A Foundation for Clinical Neuroscience*, 2nd ed.; McGraw-Hill Medical: New York, NY, USA, 2009.
25. Biederman, J.; Faraone, S.V. Current concepts on the neurobiology of Attention-Deficit/Hyperactivity Disorder. *J. Atten. Disord.* **2002**, *6*, 7–16. [CrossRef]
26. Bidwell, L.C.; McClernon, F.J.; Kollins, S.H. Cognitive enhancers for the treatment of ADHD. *Pharmacol. Biochem. Behav.* **2011**, *99*, 262–274. [CrossRef] [PubMed]
27. Cortese, S. The neurobiology and genetics of attention-deficit/hyperactivity disorder (ADHD): What every clinician should know. *Eur. J. Paediatr. Neurol.* **2012**, *16*, 422–433. [CrossRef] [PubMed]
28. Lesch, K.P.; Merker, S.; Reif, A.; Novak, M. Dances with black widow spiders: Dysregulation of glutamate signalling enters centre stage in ADHD. *Eur. Neuropsychopharmacol.* **2013**, *23*, 479–491. [CrossRef]
29. Gizer, I.R.; Ficks, C.; Waldman, I.D. Candidate gene studies of ADHD: A meta-analytic review. *Hum. Genet.* **2009**, *126*, 51–90. [CrossRef]
30. Kebir, O.; Joober, R. Neuropsychological endophenotypes in attention-deficit/hyperactivity disorder: A review of genetic association studies. *Eur. Arch. Psychiatry Clin. Neurosci.* **2011**, *261*, 583–594. [CrossRef] [PubMed]
31. Berry, M.D. The potential of trace amines and their receptors for treating neurological and psychiatric diseases. *Rev. Recent Clin. Trials.* **2007**, *2*, 3–19. [CrossRef]
32. Sotnikova, T.D.; Caron, M.G.; Gainetdinov, R.R. Trace amine-associated receptors as emerging therapeutic targets. *Mol. Pharmacol.* **2009**, *76*, 229–235. [PubMed]

33. Chandler, D.J.; Waterhouse, B.D.; Gao, W.J. New perspectives on catecholaminergic regulation of executive circuits: Evidence for independent modulation of prefrontal functions by midbrain dopaminergic and noradrenergic neurons. *Front. Neural Circuits* **2014**, *8*, 53. [CrossRef] [PubMed]
34. Rahi, V.; Kumar, P. Animal models of attention-deficit hyperactivity disorder (ADHD). *Int. J. Dev. Neurosci.* **2021**, *81*, 107–124. [CrossRef]
35. Russell, V.A. Hypodopaminergic and hypernoradrenergic activity in prefrontal cortex slices of an animal model for attention-deficit hyperactivity disorder—The spontaneously hypertensive rat. *Behav. Brain Res.* **2002**, *130*, 191–196. [CrossRef]
36. Matias, A.; Zimmer, F.J.; Lorenzen, A.; Keil, R.; Schwabe, U. Affinity of central adenosine A_1 receptors is decreased in spontaneously hypertensive rats. *Eur. J. Pharmacol.* **1993**, *244*, 223–230. [CrossRef]
37. Fredholm, B.B.; Bättig, K.; Holmén, J.; Nehlig, A.; Zvartau, E.E. Actions of Caffeine in the Brain with Special Reference to Factors That Contribute to Its Widespread Use. *Pharmacol. Rev.* **1999**, *51*, 83–133.
38. Latini, S.; Pedata, F. Adenosine in the central nervous system: Release mechanisms and extracellular concentrations. *J. Neurochem.* **2001**, *79*, 463–484. [CrossRef]
39. Ferré, S. An update on the mechanisms of the psychostimulant effects of caffeine. *J. Neurochem.* **2008**, *105*, 1067–1079. [CrossRef]
40. Chen, Y.; Parrish, T.B. Caffeine dose effect on activation-induced BOLD and CBF responses. *Neuroimage* **2009**, *46*, 577–583. [CrossRef]
41. Diukova, A.; Ware, J.; Smith, J.E.; Evans, C.J.; Murphy, K.; Rogers, P.J.; Wise, R.G. Separating neural and vascular effects of caffeine using simultaneous EEG-FMRI: Differential effects of caffeine on cognitive and sensorimotor brain responses. *Neuroimage* **2012**, *62*, 239–249. [CrossRef] [PubMed]
42. Garfinkel, B.D.; Webster, C.D.; Sloman, L. Responses to methylphenidate and varied doses of caffeine in children with attention deficit disorder. *Can. J. Psychiatry* **1981**, *26*, 395–401.
43. Firestone, P.; Davey, J.; Goodman, J.T.; Peters, S. The effects of caffeine and methylphenidate on hyperactive children. *J. Am. Acad. Child Psychiatry* **1978**, *17*, 445–456. [CrossRef]
44. Cunha, R.A.; Ferré, S.; Vaugeois, J.M.; Chen, J.F. Potential therapeutic interest of adenosine A_{2A} receptors in psychiatric disorders. *Curr. Pharm. Des.* **2008**, *14*, 1512–1524. [CrossRef]
45. Cunha, R.A. How does adenosine control neuronal dysfunction and neurodegeneration? *J. Neurochem.* **2016**, *139*, 1019–1055. [CrossRef] [PubMed]
46. Harvey, D.H.; Marsh, R.W. The effects of de-caffeinated coffee versus whole coffee on hyperactive children. *Dev. Med. Child Neurol.* **1978**, *20*, 81–86. [CrossRef]
47. Huestis, R.; Arnold, L.; Smeltzer, D. Caffeine versus methylphenidate and d-amphetamine in minimal brain dysfunction: A double-blind comparison. *Am. J. Psychiatry* **1975**, *132*, 868–870. [PubMed]
48. Garfinkel, B.D.; Webster, C.D.; Sloman, L. Individual responses to methylphenidate and caffeine in children with minimal brain dysfunction. *Can. Med. Assoc. J.* **1975**, *113*, 729–732.
49. Marmorstein, N.R. Energy drink and coffee consumption and psychopathology symptoms among early adolescents: Crosssectional and longitudinal associations. *J. Caffeine Res.* **2016**, *6*, 64–72. [CrossRef]
50. Moher, D.; Liberati, A.; Tetzlaff, J.; Altman, D.G.; The PRISMA Group. Preferred Reporting Items for Systematic Reviews and Meta-Analyses: The PRISMA Statement. *PLoS Med.* **2009**, *6*, e1000097. [CrossRef] [PubMed]
51. Pandolfo, P.; Machado, N.J.; Köfalvi, A.; Takahashi, R.N.; Cunha, R.A. Caffeine regulates frontocorticostriatal dopamine transporter density and improves attention and cognitive deficits in an animal model of attention deficit hyperactivity disorder. *Eur. Neuropsychopharmacol.* **2013**, *23*, 317–328. [CrossRef]
52. Ouchi, H.; Ono, K.; Murakami, Y.; Matsumoto, K. Social isolation induces deficit of latent learning performance in mice: A putative animal model of attention deficit/hyperactivity disorder. *Behav. Brain. Res.* **2013**, *238*, 146–153. [CrossRef]
53. Caballero, M.; Núñez, F.; Ahern, S.; Cuffí, M.L.; Carbonell, L.; Sánchez, S.; Fernández-Dueñas, V.; Ciruela, F. Caffeine improves attention deficit in neonatal 6-OHDA lesioned rats, an animal model of attention deficit hyperactivity disorder (ADHD). *Neurosci. Lett.* **2011**, *494*, 44–48. [CrossRef]
54. Ruiz-Oliveira, J.; Silva, P.F.; Luchiari, A.C. Coffee time: Low caffeine dose promotes attention and focus in zebrafish. *Learn. Behav.* **2019**, *47*, 227–233. [CrossRef]
55. Higgins, G.A.; Grzelak, M.E.; Pond, A.J.; Cohen-Williams, M.E.; Hodgson, R.A.; Varty, G.B. The effect of caffeine to increase reaction time in the rat during a test of attention is mediated through antagonism of adenosine A2A receptors. *Behav. Brain. Res.* **2007**, *185*, 32–42. [CrossRef] [PubMed]
56. França, A.P.; Schamne, M.G.; de Souza, B.S.; da Luz Scheffer, D.; Bernardelli, A.K.; Corrêa, T.; de Souza Izídio, G.; Latini, A.; da Silva-Santos, J.E.; Canas, P.M.; et al. Caffeine consumption plus physical exercise improves behavioral impairments and stimulates neuroplasticity in Spontaneously Hypertensive Rats (SHR): An animal model of attention deficit hyperactivity disorder. *Mol. Neurobiol.* **2020**, *57*, 3902–3919. [CrossRef]
57. Nunes, F.; Pochmann, D.; Almeida, A.S.; Marques, D.M.; Porciúncula, L.O. Differential behavioral and biochemical responses to caffeine in male and female rats from a validated model of attention deficit and hyperactivity disorder. *Mol. Neurobiol.* **2018**, *55*, 8486–8498. [CrossRef] [PubMed]

58. Szczepanik, J.C.; de Oliveira, P.A.; de Oliveira, J.; Mack, J.M.; Engel, D.F.; Rial, D.; Moreira, E.L.; de Bem, A.F.; Prediger, R.D. Caffeine Mitigates the Locomotor Hyperactivity in Middle-aged Low-density Lipoprotein Receptor (LDLr)-Knockout Mice. *CNS Neurosci. Ther.* **2016**, *22*, 420. [CrossRef]
59. Pires, V.A.; Pamplona, F.A.; Pandolfo, P.; Prediger, R.D.S.; Takahashi, R.N. Chronic caffeine treatment during prepubertal period confers long-term cognitive benefits in adult spontaneously hypertensive rats (SHR), an animal model of attention deficit hyperactivity disorder (ADHD). *Behav. Brain. Res.* **2010**, *215*, 39–44. [CrossRef]
60. Prediger, R.D.S.; Pamplona, F.A.; Fernandes, D.; Takahashi, R.N. Caffeine improves spatial learning deficits in an animal model of attention deficit hyperactivity disorder (ADHD)-the spontaneously hypertensive rat (SHR). *Int. J. Neuropsychopharmacol.* **2005**, *8*, 583–594. [CrossRef] [PubMed]
61. Leffa, D.T.; Ferreira, S.G.; Machado, N.J.; Souza, C.M.; Rosa, F.D.; de Carvalho, C.; Kincheski, G.C.; Takahashi, R.N.; Porciúncula, L.O.; Souza, D.O. Caffeine and cannabinoid receptors modulate impulsive behavior in an animal model of attentional deficit and hyperactivity disorder. *Eur. J. Neurosci.* **2019**, *49*, 1673–1683. [CrossRef] [PubMed]
62. Pires, V.A.; Pamplona, F.A.; Pandolfo, P.; Fernandes, D.; Prediger, R.D.; Takahashi, R.N. Adenosine receptor antagonists improve short-term object-recognition ability of spontaneously hypertensive rats: A rodent model of attention-deficit hyperactivity disorder. *Behav. Pharmacol.* **2009**, *20*, 134–145. [CrossRef]
63. Alves, C.B.; Almeida, A.S.; Marques, D.M.; Faé, A.H.L.; Machado, A.C.L.; Oliveira, D.L.; Porciúncula, L.O. Caffeine and adenosine A_{2A} receptors rescue neuronal development in vitro of frontal cortical neurons in a rat model of attention deficit and hyperactivity disorder. *Neuropharmacology* **2020**, *166*, 107782. [CrossRef] [PubMed]
64. Leon, M.R. Effects of caffeine on cognitive, psychomotor, and affective performance of children with attention-deficit/hyperactivity disorder. *J. Atten. Disord.* **2000**, *4*, 27–47. [CrossRef]
65. Ioannidis, K.; Chamberlain, S.R.; Müller, U. Ostracising caffeine from the pharmacological arsenal for attention-deficit hyperactivity disorder—Was this a correct decision? A literature review. *J. Psychopharmacol.* **2014**, *28*, 830–836. [CrossRef]
66. Fredholm, B.B. Adenosine and neuroprotection. *Int. Rev. Neurobiol.* **1996**, *40*, 259–280.
67. Claghorn, G.C.; Thompson, Z.; Wi, K.; Van, L.; Garland, T., Jr. Caffeine stimulates voluntary wheel running in mice without increasing aerobic capacity. *Physiol. Behav.* **2017**, *170*, 133–140. [CrossRef]
68. Cunha, R.A.; Agostinho, P.M. Chronic caffeine consumption prevents memory disturbance in different animal models of memory decline. *J. Alzheimers Dis.* **2010**, *20*, 95–116. [CrossRef]

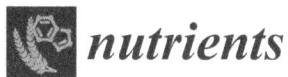

Review

Diet and Anxiety: A Scoping Review

Monique Aucoin [1,*], Laura LaChance [2,3], Umadevi Naidoo [4,5], Daniella Remy [1,6], Tanisha Shekdar [1], Negin Sayar [1], Valentina Cardozo [1], Tara Rawana [1], Irina Chan [1] and Kieran Cooley [1,7,8,9]

[1] Canadian College of Naturopathic Medicine, Toronto, ON M2K 1E2, Canada; dremy@ndnet.ccnm.edu (D.R.); tshekdar@ndnet.ccnm.edu (T.S.); sayar.negin@gmail.com (N.S.); valentinacardozov@gmail.com (V.C.); trawana@ndnet.ccnm.edu (T.R.); irinacchan@gmail.com (I.C.); kcooley@ccnm.edu (K.C.)
[2] Department of Psychiatry, McGill University, Montreal, QC H3A 0G4, Canada; laura.lachance@mail.mcgill.ca
[3] St. Mary's Hospital Centre, Montreal, QC H3T 1M5, Canada
[4] Massachusetts General Hospital, Boston, MA 02114, USA; unaidoo@mgh.harvard.edu
[5] Department of Psychiatry, Harvard Medical School, Boston, MA 02115, USA
[6] Anthrophi Technologies, Toronto, ON M6H1W2, Canada
[7] School of Public Health, Australian Research Centre in Complementary and Integrative Medicine (ARCCIM), University of Technology Sydney, Ultimo 2007, Australia
[8] Pacific College of Health Sciences, San Diego, CA 92108, USA
[9] National Centre for Naturopathic Medicine, Southern Cross University, Lismore 2480, Australia
* Correspondence: maucoin@ccnm.edu

Abstract: Anxiety disorders are the most common group of mental disorders. There is mounting evidence demonstrating the importance of nutrition in the development and progression of mental disorders such as depression; however, less is known about the role of nutrition in anxiety disorders. This scoping review sought to systematically map the existing literature on anxiety disorders and nutrition in order to identify associations between dietary factors and anxiety symptoms or disorder prevalence as well as identify gaps and opportunities for further research. The review followed established methodological approaches for scoping reviews. Due to the large volume of results, an online program (Abstrackr) with artificial intelligence features was used. Studies reporting an association between a dietary constituent and anxiety symptoms or disorders were counted and presented in figures. A total of 55,914 unique results were identified. After a full-text review, 1541 articles met criteria for inclusion. Analysis revealed an association between less anxiety and more fruits and vegetables, omega-3 fatty acids, "healthy" dietary patterns, caloric restriction, breakfast consumption, ketogenic diet, broad-spectrum micronutrient supplementation, zinc, magnesium and selenium, probiotics, and a range of phytochemicals. Analysis revealed an association between higher levels of anxiety and high-fat diet, inadequate tryptophan and dietary protein, high intake of sugar and refined carbohydrates, and "unhealthy" dietary patterns. Results are limited by a large percentage of animal and observational studies. Only 10% of intervention studies involved participants with anxiety disorders, limiting the applicability of the findings. High quality intervention studies involving participants with anxiety disorders are warranted.

Keywords: nutrition; diet; food; anxiety; mental health; psychiatry; nutritional science; dietetics

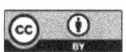

1. Introduction

The term anxiety describes the experience of worry, apprehension, or nervousness in association with physical, cognitive, and behavioral symptoms. Anxiety may be experienced occasionally as part of normal life and may be adaptive if it increases preparedness for novel situations. If anxiety symptoms are persistent, excessive, or interfere with functioning, they can become pathological [1].

Several anxiety disorders have been defined. Generalized anxiety disorder involves excessive worry in multiple domains and associated physical symptoms that are present for at least six months leading to clinically significant distress or impairment in functioning [1].

Panic disorder is characterized by unexpected and recurrent panic attacks and at least one month of persistent worry about having a subsequent panic attack or significant behavior changes related to the attack [2]. Agoraphobia involves feelings of intense fear of situations or spaces where escape may be difficult or help may not be available in the event or panic or other incapacitating symptoms [3]. Social anxiety disorder involves marked anxiety and fear of a social situation where an individual is exposed to possible scrutiny by others [4]. Specific phobia is an excessive fear of specific object or situation [5].

Anxiety disorders exert a significant burden at both an individual and societal level. Individuals with anxiety disorders report a high degree of psychological distress, significant disability [6] and a reduction in quality of life [7]. The presence of an anxiety disorder is associated with higher use of both primary care, emergency room visits, and specialist healthcare services [8]. These disorders are also highly prevalent. The national comorbidities study established the lifetime prevalence of any anxiety disorder at 31.2%, the highest of any category of psychiatric illnesses [9].

The treatment approaches most frequently used in the management of anxiety disorders are psychotherapy and psychopharmacology [10]. While many patients find these therapies beneficial, a significant number of individuals report that these treatment options are not accessible, tolerable, or effective in providing adequate relief of anxiety symptoms [11]. For these reasons, there is interest in the evaluation of adjunctive or alternative therapeutic approaches.

Nutritional psychiatry is an emerging field of study related to the use of nutritional interventions in the prevention and treatment of mental health disorders. Despite increasing evidence of beneficial effects, nutritional recommendations are provided to psychiatric patients infrequently in clinical practice. Recently, high quality intervention studies have demonstrated an antidepressant effect of nutritional interventions [12,13]. However, the amount of research on anxiety disorders lags behind that of mood disorders [14,15]. There is a clear lack of studies delivering diet counselling, education, or food as an intervention to individuals with diagnosed anxiety disorders as well as systematic synthesis of the existing literature on the relationship between dietary factors and anxiety symptoms or disorders. The objective of the present review was to systematically map out the body of existing literature on anxiety symptoms/disorders and nutrition in order to identify nutritional factors associated with higher or lower levels of anxiety and to identify knowledge gaps and opportunities for further research.

2. Materials and Methods

The review followed established methodological approaches for scoping reviews using the framework presented by Arskey and O'Malley for the conduct of scoping reviews [16]. Scoping reviews aim to identify and describe the breadth of literature on a topic when it is either highly complex, involves a broad array of study designs, or when a comprehensive review is being completed for the first time; all of these factors apply to the present review. Scoping reviews aim to map key concepts in a field of study and the available types of evidence. The review is completed in a way that is systematic, highly rigorous, and transparent in order to minimize bias. The protocol used in the present study was adapted from a similar project completed by the authors on the topic of diet and psychosis [17].

An extensive *a priori* search strategy was developed and executed with the guidance of an experienced medical librarian. Using the Ovid platform, we searched Ovid MEDLINE®, including Epub Ahead of Print, In-Process & Other Non-Indexed Citations, and Embase Classic + Embase. We used controlled vocabulary (e.g., "Anxiety Disorders", "Nutritional Physiological Phenomena", "Food") and keywords (e.g., anxiety, nutrition, diet). We adjusted vocabulary and syntax as necessary across the databases. There were no language or date restrictions on any of the searches, but we removed opinion pieces (e.g., editorials) from the results. We performed the searches on 25 March 2020. The full search, as executed, is available in Supplemental File S1.

Screening of abstracts and titles was completed using the online open-source program Abstrackr [18] which allowed for concurrent and blind duplicate screening as well as tagging by dietary constituent. Manual screening was completed until the program's artificial intelligence predicted the presence of additional relevant studies as unlikely. Previous testing of this program has demonstrated that the likelihood of missing relevant studies is very low [18–20]. As an extra precaution, once screening had reached the point where Abstrackr's prediction score reported 'zero additional studies likely to be relevant', and no studies were being identified as being relevant, an additional 100 articles were screened in each section before screening was stopped. Screening of abstracts and titles was completed in duplicate. Disagreement was resolved by consensus.

Studies were eligible for inclusion if they involved the evaluation of changes in the level of anxiety symptoms or the presence/absence of anxiety disorders in humans or animal models as well as assessing or modifying a component of participant diet. This included assessment or modification of dietary patterns, individual foods, supplements, or natural health products that provide an active constituent naturally occurring in the general North American diet. Studies were ineligible if they assessed or administered herbal medicines (apart from those used for culinary purposes in the general North American diet) or constituents which are not typically found in significant quantities in the human diet (i.e., St. John's Wort, GABA, or S-adenosylmethionine) or if they assessed levels of endogenously produced dietary components (i.e., cholesterol, vitamin D, or non-essential amino acids) in the absence of supplementation or measurement of intake. Eligible study designs included human observational and experimental studies, animal studies, and meta-analyses. Studies were excluded if they assessed the impact of maternal diet on offspring anxiety levels. Review articles, opinion papers, letters, and systematic reviews (without meta-analysis) were excluded, as were non-English language papers or inaccessible papers in cases where the abstract contained insufficient information for data extraction.

Full text screening was completed concurrently with data extraction. Data extraction was completed using piloted extraction templates developed for a similar scoping review conducted by the study authors and double checked by MA for accuracy [17]. Analysis was completed by sorting the studies with common interventions and methodology types and counting the number of studies reporting an association with increased or decreased anxiety symptoms/disorders, or no association. These data were used to create figures that communicate an overview of the evidence on each topic. Studies reporting a statistically significant improvement in at least one subpopulation or measure of anxiety symptomatology were categorized as "associated with decreased anxiety". Studies reporting an increase in anxiety symptoms or prevalence in at least one subpopulation or measure of anxiety symptomatology were categorized as "associated with increased anxiety". Studies that reported no significant change in anxiety symptoms or prevalence were categorized as "no association with anxiety". A small number of studies which reported mixed findings such as a combination of increased and decreased anxiety symptoms were not included in the figures. In order to allow concise display and the comparison of all studies, the number of studies reporting an association between improved symptoms with higher intake of a nutrient were combined with studies reporting and association between worse symptoms with lower intake of the nutrient. Counts are depicted in figures. The figures are oriented so that they report the relationship between higher intake of the diet constituent with anxiety. Within each section, a narrative summary was completed to highlight trends, gaps, and areas that warrant further study. When available, narrative summaries also reported on proposed mechanisms and safety. Finally, we created a list of dietary factors that, based on the review findings, may to be associated with less anxiety and more anxiety symptoms/disorders. This process of categorization was done based on the following criteria related to the volume and consistency of evidence. Dietary factors were included in these two categories when there were at least five studies reporting on the relationship with anxiety, and the majority of the data points (>60%) showed a consistent association.

These criteria were developed post hoc as the volume, and consistency of the evidence was unknown at the time of protocol development.

3. Results

3.1. Search Results

The search identified 55,914 unique results that were screened in two phases: by title/abstract and by full text. The study authors manually screened 13,286 results while Abstrackr's artificial intelligence screened the remaining results. Following title and abstract screening, 2213 articles were included.

Seventeen articles could not be retrieved in full text. During full text screening, an additional 655 studies were excluded (Supplemental File S2). 1541 studies were included in the final data analysis (Figure 1, Supplemental File S3).

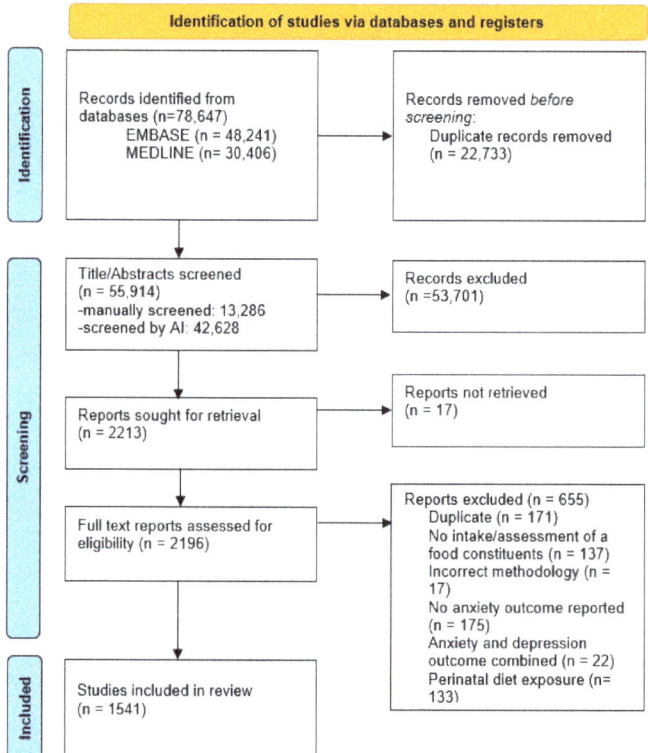

Figure 1. PRISMA flow diagram. AI: artificial intelligence.

3.2. Study Characteristics

More than half of the studies in our analysis were conducted using animal models (*n* = 859) (Figure 2). The animal studies were primarily conducted in rodents (97%) with the remaining 3% of studies conducted in zebrafish, pigs, lemurs, monkeys, cats, horses, and tilapia.

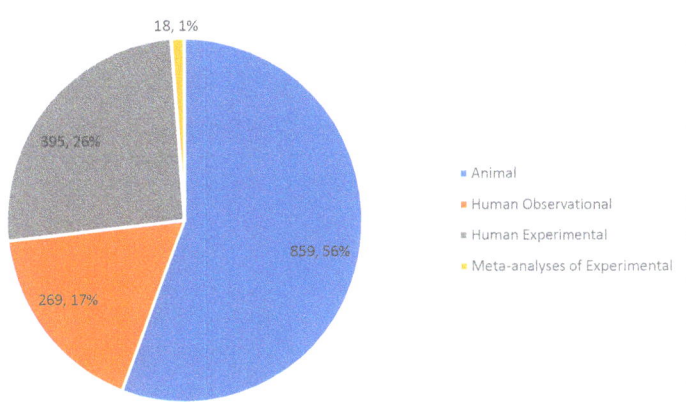

Figure 2. Distribution of included studies by methodology (count, percent).

The observational studies included 14 case reports; in 11 reports, subjects had anxiety disorders or elevated anxiety symptoms at baseline (Figure 3). In total, the reports described 44 individual cases. An additional 255 publications described cross-sectional, prospective, or retrospective observational studies. One meta-analysis of observational studies was conducted [21]. Of the observational studies, 88% were cross-sectional in design and 13 studies (5%) specifically included individuals with anxiety disorders or elevated anxiety symptoms. Nutrient intake was assessed in 201 studies while nutrient levels, in various body tissues, were measured in 40 studies. Sample size varied widely, from 14 to 296,121 participants (Mean: 6315.7, SD: 28,423.9).

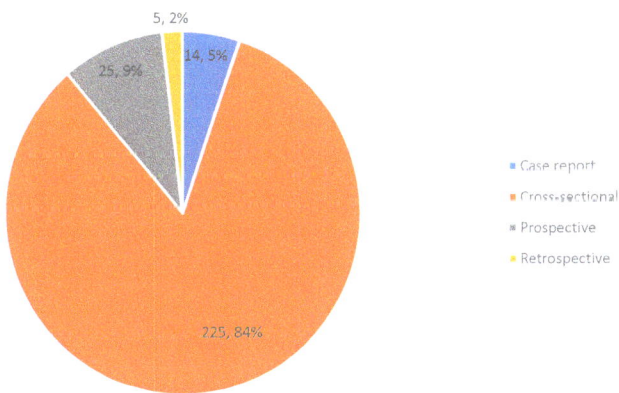

Figure 3. Types of observational studies (count, percent).

Regarding experimental studies, 395 met criteria for inclusion as well as an additional 18 meta-analyses of experimental studies. Of the individual studies, the number of participants ranged from 3 to 2730 (Mean: 99.3, SD: 198.3). Of the 395 trials, 335 (85%) included a comparison arm, 312 (79%) utilized randomization, and 23 (61%) utilized blinding. Thirty-nine trials (10%) included participants with anxiety disorders or elevated anxiety symptoms. An additional 57 trials assessed anxiety in participants with other psychiatric illnesses while the remaining studies included participants with medical illnesses or healthy participants (Figure 4). Excluding the studies that assessed the immediate impact of food on anxiety symptoms ($n = 72$), the average duration of the experimental studies was 15.8 weeks (SD: 18.3 weeks). Most of the studies ($n = 331$) provided the dietary intervention without co-interventions. An exercise co-intervention was delivered in 32 studies, while 20 included a psychosocial component and ten co-administered a medication. Sixty-nine percent of experimental studies identified a primary outcome related to mental health.

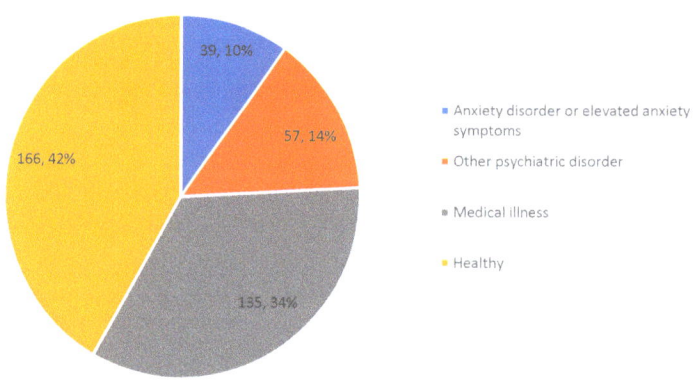

Figure 4. Participant populations in human experimental studies (count, percent).

3.3. Dietary Patterns

Many studies were identified that assessed the impact of dietary patterns on anxiety symptoms severity or anxiety disorder prevalence including both animal models ($n = 101$) and human studies with observational ($n = 102$) and experimental ($n = 84$) designs. Dietary pattern studies evaluated the impact of combinations of foods or patterns of eating. Studies looked at both the types of foods that were consumed (Figure 5) and the quantity and timing of food consumption (Figure 6). Because studies may have defined specific dietary patterns differently, it is noted that significant heterogeneity exists within each category. In general, "Healthy" diet patterns were described as diets aligned with generally accepted principles of healthy eating. Many involved the calculation of a healthy eating score or index and were defined by higher intake of vegetables, fruit, whole grains, fish, legumes, and unprocessed meat. Diets or dietary patterns defined as "Unhealthy" or "Western" generally included higher intake of processed foods, sugar and sweetened foods, soft drinks, fried foods, processed meats, "junk food", and "fast food". In the animal studies, the "Western" or "Cafeteria" diet included a combination of high fat and high carbohydrate, in particular, high saturated fat and high refined carbohydrates. In many cases, the diet was designed to be highly palatable and to induce obesity [22,23].

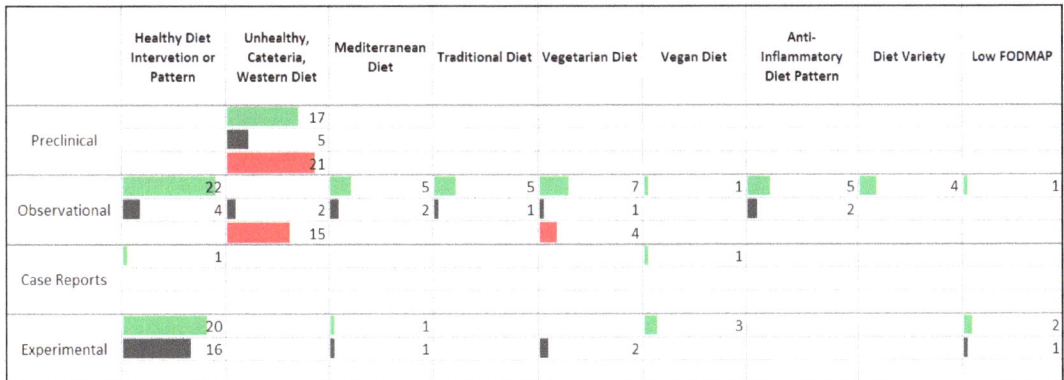

Figure 5. Studies assessing the composition of dietary patterns. ■ Higher intake or levels associated with decreased anxiety. ■ No association between intake or levels and anxiety. ■ Higher intake or levels associated with increased anxiety.

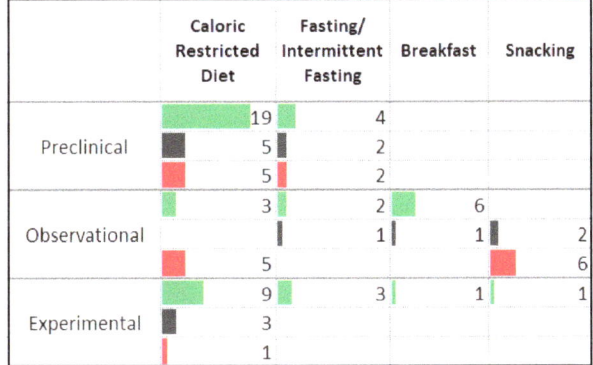

Figure 6. Studies assessing the amount of food consumed or timing of eating. ■ Higher intake or levels associated with decreased anxiety. ■ No association between intake or levels and anxiety. ■ Higher intake or levels associated with increased anxiety.

The animal studies reported a mixture of anxiogenic and anxiolytic effects following administration of the "unhealthy", "cafeteria", or "Western" style eating patterns. Predominantly anxiolytic effects were seen following caloric restriction and fasting.

Observational studies showed an association between lower anxiety symptom severity or disorder prevalence and "healthy" diet patterns, the Mediterranean diet, traditional diets, the vegetarian diet, consumption of breakfast, anti-inflammatory diet patterns, and increased diet variety. Higher anxiety symptom severity or disorder prevalence was associated with "unhealthy" diet patterns, caloric restriction, and snacking. It is noted that among the observational studies assessing the relationship between vegetarianism and anxiety symptoms, two of the three studies that reported an increase in anxiety were prospective in design while all of the studies reporting an association between the diet pattern and less anxiety were cross-sectional in design. Two case reports described improvement in anxiety symptom severity following multimodal interventions with a dietary component. One involved the elimination of "inflammatory foods" in combination with exercise and psychological treatment [24]. The other delivered a vegan diet in combination with fruit and vegetable juice, nutritional supplements, exercise and stress management techniques [25].

Of the experimental studies delivering an intervention that promoted healthy eating behaviors, twenty reported a reduction in anxiety symptoms while sixteen did not observe a significant effect. Only two of these trials recruited individuals with anxiety disorders [26,27]; the remaining studies recruited individuals with medical illnesses or healthy participants. One randomized controlled trial enrolled participants with moderate to severe anxiety disorders and assessed the impact of dietary counselling, in combination with a multivitamin and a herbal remedy, compared to a psychosocial intervention, and reported a significant improvement in anxiety symptoms with the combination intervention as compared to the psychosocial intervention [26]. Another study randomized individuals with anxiety and/or depressive disorders to either dietician consultations or an attention control intervention; significant improvement was seen in both treatment groups [27]. Nine of thirteen studies promoting caloric restriction reported an improvement in anxiety symptoms. While one of the studies recruited participants with elevated anxiety symptoms [28], all involved overweight and obese participants. A meta-analysis of studies delivering caloric restriction to adults with obesity did not find a significant reduction in anxiety symptoms [29] while a meta-analysis on the same topic that included child and adolescent populations did report a reduction in anxiety [30].

3.4. Carbohydrates

One trend that was observed among the carbohydrate studies was a relationship between higher intake of simple or refined carbohydrates, higher glycemic index diet, or sugar intake, and higher levels of anxiety (Figure 7). This association was reported by several animal and observational studies. Similarly, 75% of the 12 animal studies and the only human experimental trial assessing the impact of artificial sweeteners (aspartame, saccharin, and sorbitol) reported an increase in anxiety symptoms. One observational study reported on the relationship between fiber and anxiety; at long term follow up two to three years after completing a program aimed at increasing fiber intake, 14 irritable bowel syndrome patients reported lower anxiety symptoms [31].

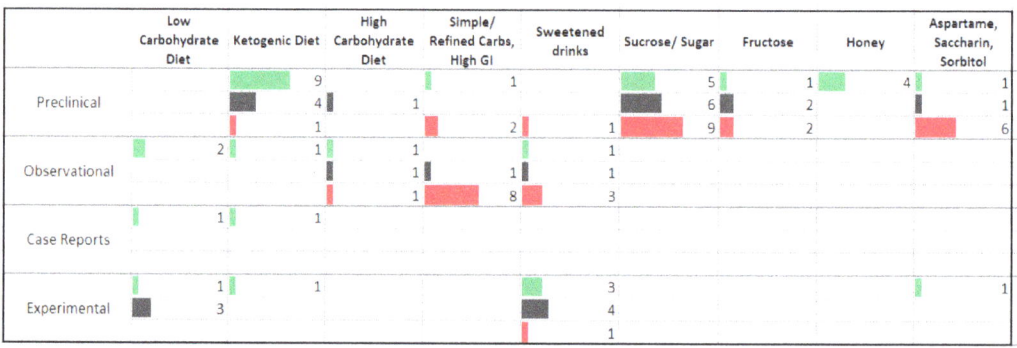

Figure 7. Studies assessing dietary carbohydrates and anxiety. ■ Higher intake or levels associated with decreased anxiety. ■ No association between intake or levels and anxiety. ■ Higher intake or levels associated with increased anxiety.

Very limited research has been undertaken in the form of human experimental studies that sought to reduce carbohydrate intake ($n = 4$); none included participants with anxiety disorders. Of four studies, one study involving obese or overweight participants reported an improvement in anxiety symptoms following a low carbohydrate diet. Eight studies evaluated the effect of consuming sweetened drinks on anxiety in humans. These studies administered carbohydrate-rich drinks to patients undergoing surgical procedures and measured the immediate effects on anxiety symptom severity, often in comparison with pre-operative fasting. The findings of these studies were mixed.

3.5. Protein

Limited research has investigated the effects of different levels of dietary protein on anxiety symptom severity or disorder prevalence (Figure 8). Two thirds of the 12 animal studies assessing the impact of protein malnutrition reported a worsening of anxiety symptoms. Four human experimental studies delivered a high protein diet; three studies, involving participants without anxiety disorders, reported no effect on anxiety symptom severity. One experimental study involving three participants with elevated anxiety symptoms reported improvement following a high protein, low carbohydrate diet [32]. A very small amount of research has been completed comparing plant and animal sources of protein. One observational study reported a benefit with higher intake of animal protein [33], the other reported no difference [34]. The food additive monosodium glutamate (MSG), a modified amino acid, was associated with increased levels of anxiety in animal models.

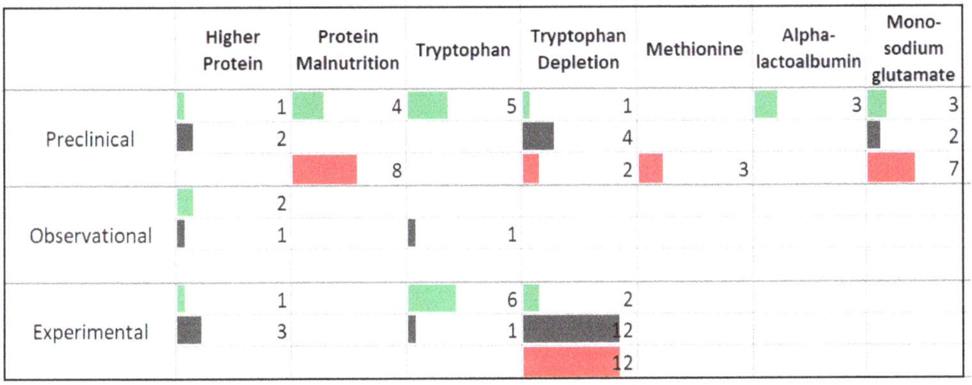

	Higher Protein	Protein Malnutrition	Tryptophan	Tryptophan Depletion	Methionine	Alpha-lactoalbumin	Mono-sodium glutamate
Preclinical	1	4	5	1		3	3
	2			4			2
		8		2	3		7
Observational		2					
		1		1			
Experimental		1		6	2		
		3		1	2		
				12			

Figure 8. Studies assessing protein and anxiety. ■ Higher intake or levels associated with decreased anxiety. ■ No association between intake or levels and anxiety. ■ Higher intake or levels associated with increased anxiety.

There was an association between higher anxiety symptoms and tryptophan depletion, among human experimental studies. Supplementation of tryptophan resulted in decreased anxiety symptoms in both animal and experimental studies. Of the studies assessing the effect of tryptophan depletion, 10 involved individuals with anxiety disorders; five reported no effect while five reported a worsening of anxiety symptoms. Of the studies administering a tryptophan supplement, two involved individuals with anxiety disorders [35,36]; both studies reported improvement.

3.6. Fats

Compared with other categories of nutrients, a large number of animal studies have investigated the effects of increased intake of fat on rodent models of anxiety (Figure 9). Many animal studies ($n = 39$) have reported an anxiogenic effect of a high fat diet. A smaller number have reported a similar effect from diets high in cholesterol ($n = 5$) and trans fats ($n = 6$). A large number of animal studies have reported anxiolytic effects of omega-3 fatty acids ($n = 35$), Docosahexaenoic acid ($n = 9$), Eicosapentaenoic acid ($n = 3$), and alpha-linolenic acid ($n = 4$). Human observational studies reported an association between higher intake of omega-3 fatty acids and lower levels of anxiety.

	Dietary Fish	Nuts and Seeds	Fish Oil, EPA or DHA	ALA/ flaxseed oil	Omega-6, Omega-3+6	Omega-9/ oleic acid/ MUFAs	High Fat Diet	Low Fat Diet	High Cholesterol Diet	Trans Fat	Saturated/ Animal Fat	Phospholipids
Preclinical		4	49	4	3	2	14				1	2
		1	15	2	4		10			1	1	1
			3	1	2		39		5	5	3	
Observational	3	1	11	1	3	3						
	4		1		1		1				2	
			3		3	2	1	1		1	3	
Experimental	1		11		1	3		1			1	
	1		11		1			4			1	2

Figure 9. Studies assessing dietary fats and anxiety. ■ Higher intake or levels associated with decreased anxiety. ■ No association between intake or levels and anxiety. ■ Higher intake or levels associated with increased anxiety.

Twenty-two human experimental studies have measured changes in anxiety symptoms following supplementation with omega-3 fatty acids. Eleven studies reported an improvement in anxiety symptoms, the remaining studies were equivocal. Two of three meta-analyses of trials delivering omega-3 fatty acid supplements reported benefit to anxiety symptoms [37–39]. While nine of the experimental studies included participants with psychiatric disorders such as eating disorders, substance use disorders and ADHD, only one trial involved participants with anxiety disorders [40]. In this trial, researchers provided polyunsaturated fatty acids (omega-3 and omega-6) to 126 sufferers of test anxiety and reported an improvement in symptom severity after three weeks.

3.7. Vitamins

A large number of animal studies (n = 56) have investigated the effects of vitamins B, C, D, E, choline, and folic acid and reported primarily anxiolytic effects (Figure 10). Among the human observational studies, the majority of studies assessing vitamin C, vitamin E, and broad-spectrum micronutrients reported an association with less anxiety symptoms while the majority of the studies assessing levels or intake of B vitamins and folic acid reported no association with anxiety symptom severity. Additionally, five case reports reported improvement in anxiety symptoms following broad-spectrum micronutrient supplementation.

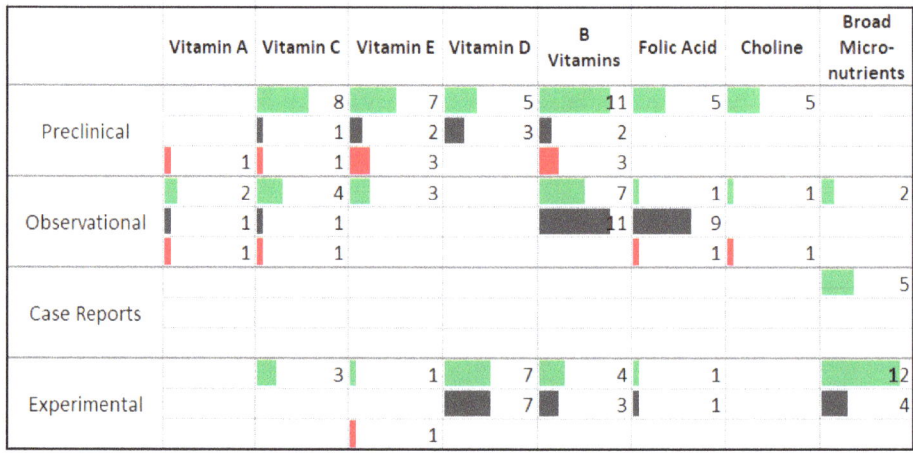

	Vitamin A	Vitamin C	Vitamin E	Vitamin D	B Vitamins	Folic Acid	Choline	Broad Micro-nutrients
Preclinical		8	7	5	11	5	5	
		1	2	3	2			
	1	1		3	3			
Observational	2	4	3		7	1	1	2
	1	1			11	9		
	1	1				1	1	
Case Reports								5
Experimental		3	1	7	4	1		12
				7	3	1		4
				1				

Figure 10. Studies assessing vitamins and anxiety. ■ Higher intake or levels associated with decreased anxiety. ■ No association between intake or levels and anxiety. ■ Higher intake or levels associated with increased anxiety.

Among the human experimental studies, several studies reported improved anxiety symptoms following supplementation of vitamin C (n = 3) and broad-spectrum micronutrients (*n* = 12); mixed findings were reported by studies assessing vitamin D, B vitamins, and folic acid. Two human experimental studies involved participants with anxiety disorders. These trials delivered vitamin D [41] and two different broad-spectrum vitamin and micronutrient formulas [42], one assessed at a low and high dose. Both studies reported a reduction in anxiety symptoms.

A number of studies were identified that delivered combination natural health products to human (*n* = 22) or animal (*n* = 11) participants. The formulas included combinations of vitamins (typically two or three) or combinations of fatty acids, vitamins, minerals, probiotics, and amino acids. Among the human studies, 16 of 22 reported a significant improvement in anxiety symptoms. Among the animal studies, eight of 11 reported a significant improvement. The remaining studies reported no change. Two human trials involved participant with anxiety disorders or elevated anxiety symptoms. One included individuals with GAD [43], one included individuals with high trait anxiety levels [44]. The former delivered a combination of three vitamins (A, C, and E) and reported an improvement. The latter delivered a combination of probiotics, B vitamins and proteins and did not find a reduction in anxiety symptoms; however, other self-reported and biological markers of stress improved.

3.8. Minerals

The minerals that were assessed for an impact on anxiety symptoms in animal models most frequently are zinc, magnesium, manganese, and selenium (Figure 11). The animal studies reported a largely consistent anti-anxiety effect from supplementing these nutrients. The observational studies assessing tissue levels of magnesium most frequently reported no association with anxiety levels or anxiety disorder prevalence. Observational studies assessing tissue levels of zinc reported a combination of protective effects and no association while the observational studies assessing selenium primarily reported an association between higher intake and lower symptom severity. A small number of observational studies reported an association between higher copper or sodium and increased anxiety symptoms or disorder prevalence.

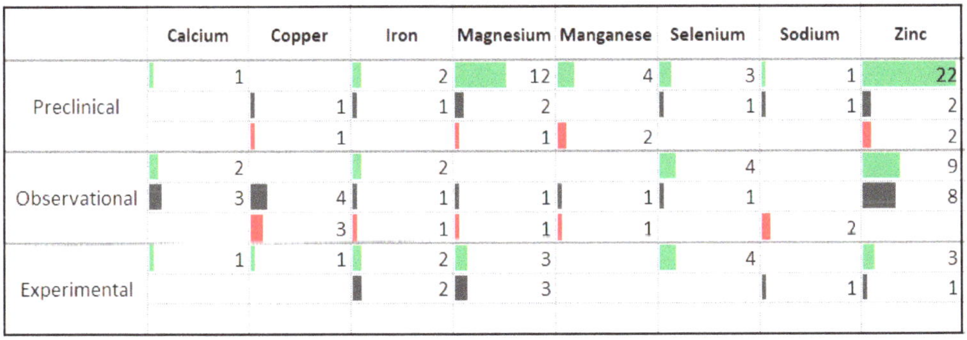

	Calcium	Copper	Iron	Magnesium	Manganese	Selenium	Sodium	Zinc
Preclinical	1			2	12	4	3	1	22
		1	1	2		1	1	2
		1		1	2			2
Observational	2		2			4		9
		3	4	1	1	1	1	8
		3	3	1	1	1	2	
Experimental	1	1		2	3		4	3
				2	3		1	1

Figure 11. Studies assessing minerals and anxiety. ■ Higher intake or levels associated with decreased anxiety. ■ No association between intake or levels and anxiety. ■ Higher intake or levels associated with increased anxiety.

A limited number of intervention studies have delivered minerals in supplemental form, including selenium, zinc, magnesium, iron, copper, and calcium. All four studies that administered selenium supplements reported improvement in anxiety symptoms. Studies administering other minerals reported a mixture of anti-anxiety effects and no effect. Only one experimental study included participants with anxiety disorders [45]. This open label study provided zinc to 38 participants for eight weeks and reported an improvement in anxiety symptoms.

3.9. Vegetables and Fruit

The results of the studies related to vegetables and fruit were largely positive (Figure 12). The majority (64%, $n = 60$) of the studies were conducted in animal models. These trials involved the administration of single fruits or vegetables and 58 of 60 reported a reduction in anxiety symptom severity. The most commonly studied foods included citrus fruits ($n = 13$), grape ($n = 7$), berries ($n = 6$), pomegranate ($n = 6$), fennel ($n = 4$), and lettuce ($n = 4$) with a wide variety of vegetables and fruits used in the remaining studies. Several observational studies reported an association between higher fruit and vegetable intake and lower levels of anxiety symptoms or disorder prevalence. A small number of intervention studies increased intake of individual vegetable or fruits; studies delivering cherries, tomato juice, orange juice, and fennel reported reduction of anxiety symptom severity. Three experimental studies delivered interventions aimed at increasing intake of vegetable and/or fruit servings consumed by participants [46–48]. Two reported a decrease in anxiety symptoms. None of the human experimental studies involved participants with anxiety disorders.

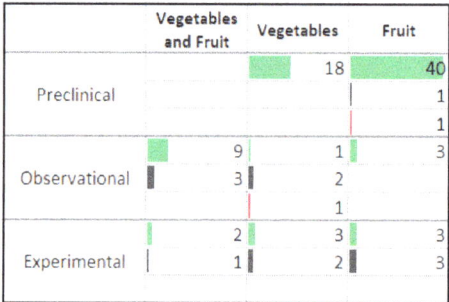

Figure 12. Studies assessing vegetables and/or fruit and anxiety. ■ Higher intake or levels associated with decreased anxiety. ■ No association between intake or levels and anxiety. ■ Higher intake or levels associated with increased anxiety.

3.10. Phytochemicals

A large number of studies have explored the effects of caffeine on anxiety symptoms (Figure 13). Many of these animal ($n = 37$) and human experimental ($n = 33$) studies administered caffeine as a supplement or provided energy drinks to subjects. While the animal studies reported a mixture of anxiogenic and anxiolytic effects, the observational and human experimental studies were more likely to report worsening anxiety symptoms with higher intake of caffeine. Several animal and human experimental studies assessed the impact of green tea and its constituents epigallocatechin-3-gallate (EGCG) and l-theanine on anxiety levels. The studies reported primarily anti-anxiety effects; however, a meta-analysis of trials delivering L-theanine and EGCG failed to detect a significant benefit [49].

Anti-anxiety effects have been reported in animal studies assessing a wide range of plants and plant constituents that may be found in the North American diet with primarily anxiolytic findings reported. These included culinary herbs (rosemary, cinnamon, coriander, basil, and nigella), herbal teas (chamomile, hibiscus, and rose tea), the phytonutrients curcumin (found in turmeric), quercetin (found in various vegetables and fruits), resveratrol (found in grapes), saffron and its constituents, soy and its constituents and other phytoestrogenic foods, nut and seed extracts, chocolate and cocoa and a variety of flavonoids, polyphenols, and carotenoids. Additionally, human experimental studies delivering green tea, curcumin, saffron, chamomile, and soy also reported anti-anxiety effects. Meta-analyses of experimental studies using chamomile [50], saffron [51], and curcumin [52,53] found a decrease in anxiety symptoms, while the meta-analysis of studies administering resveratrol reporting a non-significant improvement [54]. A small number of the human experimental studies involved participants with anxiety disorders including three studies using chamomile [55–57], two using saffron [58,59], one using curcumin [60], and one using l-theanine [61]. All trials, with the exception of the l-theanine study [61], reported a reduction in anxiety symptoms severity.

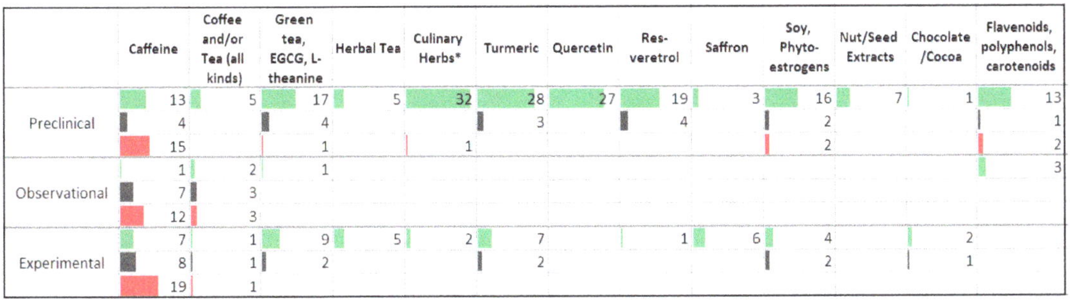

	Caffeine	Coffee and/or Tea (all kinds)	Green tea, EGCG, L-theanine	Herbal Tea	Culinary Herbs*	Turmeric	Quercetin	Resveratrol	Saffron	Soy, Phyto-estrogens	Nut/Seed Extracts	Chocolate /Cocoa	Flavenoids, polyphenols, carotenoids
Preclinical (↓)	13	5	17	5	32	28	27	19	3	16	7	1	13
Preclinical (–)	4		4			3		4		2			1
Preclinical (↑)	15		1		1					2			2
Observational (↓)	1	2	1										3
Observational (–)	7	3											
Observational (↑)	12	3											
Experimental (↓)	7	1	9	5	2	7			1	6	4		2
Experimental (–)	8	1	2			2					2		1
Experimental (↑)	19	1											

Figure 13. Studies assessing phytochemicals and anxiety * Culinary Herbs: rosemary, cinnamon, coriander, basil, nigella; Herbal tea: chamomile, hibiscus, rose tea. ■ Higher intake or levels associated with decreased anxiety. ■ No association between intake or levels and anxiety. ■ Higher intake or levels associated with increased anxiety.

3.11. Food Allergy and Intolerance

A small body of evidence, primarily observational in nature, suggests a possible connection between food allergy or intolerance and anxiety symptoms (Figure 14). Eleven of thirteen studies found higher levels of anxiety symptoms in participants with celiac disease or a food allergy. Consumption of a gluten-free diet or avoidance of other food allergens was associated with improved anxiety symptoms in observational studies and two case reports. Seven experimental studies have assessed these diet interventions with three reporting benefit. Participants were predominantly irritable bowel syndrome sufferers; none included individuals with anxiety disorders.

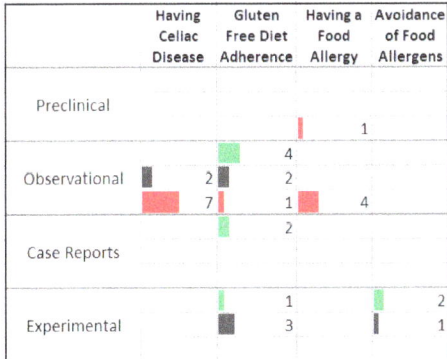

Figure 14. Studies assessing food allergies or sensitivities and anxiety. ■ Higher intake or levels associated with decreased anxiety. ■ No association between intake or levels and anxiety. ■ Higher intake or levels associated with increased anxiety.

3.12. Gut Microbiome

A number of studies have assessed the impact of probiotic and prebiotic supplementation in animals and humans (Figure 15). Animal trials have reported significant improvement in anxiety symptoms with supplementation of *Lactobacillus* strains, *Bifidobacterium* strains, combinations of *Lactobacillus* and *Bifidobacterium* strains, prebiotics, and synbiotics (combinations of prebiotics and probiotics). Interventions aimed at increasing microbiome diversity or addition of fermented foods or fiber were associated with decreased anxiety symptom severity. Administration of pathogenic organisms and antibiotics were associated with worsening anxiety symptom severity.

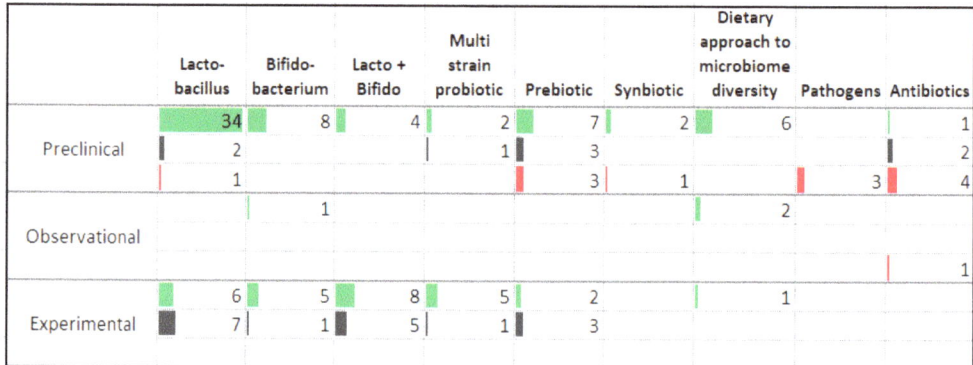

Figure 15. Studies assessing the microbiome and anxiety. ■ Higher intake or levels associated with decreased anxiety. ■ No association between intake or levels and anxiety. ■ Higher intake or levels associated with increased anxiety.

Among the human studies, predominantly positive findings were reported by trials administering *Bifidobacterium* strains and multi-strain probiotics while trials administering *Lactobacillus* strains, combinations of *Lactobacillus* and *Bifidobacterium* strains, and prebiotics reported either positive findings or no effect. Two trials involved participants with anxiety disorders [62,63]; one reported a benefit [63]. Three meta-analyses have pooled the trials assessing anxiety outcomes following probiotic supplementation [64–66]; one of three reported a significant improvement [65].

4. Discussion

The results of this scoping review suggest a possible association between more or less anxiety and a range of dietary constituents and patterns. Table 1 presents a summary of the associations identified in this review.

Table 1. Summary of nutrients and diet patterns associated with more or less anxiety symptom severity or disorder prevalence.

Association with Less Anxiety	Association with More Anxiety
• Vegetables and Fruit • Omega-3 Fatty Acids, Alpha-lipoic acid, Omega-9 Fatty acids • Nuts and seeds • "Healthy" Dietary Patterns, Mediterranean diet, Traditional Dietary Patterns, Anti-inflammatory diet pattern • Caloric Restriction • Fasting or intermittent fasting • Breakfast Consumption • Broad-Spectrum Micronutrients • Vegan Diet • Zinc, Magnesium, Selenium • Vitamin C, Vitamin E, Choline • Ketogenic Diet • Food sources of *Lactobacillus* and *Bifidobacterium* • Culinary herbs, Turmeric, Saffron, Soy, Green tea, Herbal tea, Quercetin, Resveratrol, other phytochemicals (flavonoids, polyphenols, carotenoids)	• High-fat diet, high cholesterol, high trans fat • Inadequate tryptophan and dietary protein • High intake of sugar and refined carbohydrates, artificial sweeteners • "Unhealthy" Dietary Patterns, typically defined as high in unhealthy fats and refined sugars • Snacking

4.1. Dietary Patterns

Overall, there is evidence that certain dietary patterns may influence the development and progression of anxiety disorders. The diets associated with lower anxiety include "healthy" diet patterns, the Mediterranean diet, traditional diets, the anti-inflammatory diet, and diets with increased variety. All of these diet patterns share common elements such as an emphasis on vegetables, fruit, limited sugar and refined grains, and greater consumption of minimally processed foods. However, interpretation of dietary patterns studies is somewhat hindered by the dissimilar definitions used for dietary patterns. For example, in the studies delivering "Western" style high fat/high sugar diets meant to induce obesity, a variety of dietary fats were used. The fats used to supplement some of the high fat diets included lard [67], fish oil [68], soybean oil [69] while other studies specified the percentage fat in the diet but not the type of fat that was added to achieve this amount [70–72]. Because the impact of different fatty acids on health outcomes can be highly different [73], categorizing diets as low or high in fat may result in heterogenous findings as a result of the type of fat delivered. Similarly, definitions of "healthy" diets have changed over time [74], potentially contributing to the heterogeneity of study results. Unfortunately, many studies lacked clear definitions of "healthy" or "unhealthy" diet patterns and interventions.

The outcomes associated with the vegetarian or vegan diet were generally positive although somewhat mixed and limited by being largely observational in design. The mixed findings may be due to a variety of factors. There is documentation of the adoption of a vegetarian or vegan diet following the development of an eating disorder [75]. Given the association between eating disorders and anxiety disorders [76], this may explain the association between vegetarianism and higher anxiety found in some observational studies. Furthermore, vegan diets, without adequate supplementation, may lack certain essential nutrients shown to play a role in anxiety disorders such as vitamin B12 [77] and long chain omega-3 fatty acids (EPA and DHA) [78]. Bioavailability of certain nutrients such as iron differ between plant and animal sources, possibly limiting nutrient absorption in vegan diets.

There is a significant lack of human intervention studies involving participants with anxiety disorders or elevated baseline anxiety symptoms. Many studies employed dietary patterns that were indicated for the other medical concerns of the study participants. For example, studies delivered the Low FODMAP diet to participants with irritable bowel syndrome and hypocaloric diets to participants with obesity and assessed changes in anxiety as secondary outcomes. The mechanisms by which dietary patterns impact anxiety symptoms may be the result of a combination of the mechanistic factors discussed in the following sections.

4.2. Carbohydrates

The findings of the carbohydrate studies suggest that high intake of sugar and refined carbohydrates may contribute to anxiety symptoms; however, a large proportion of trials are cross-sectional in design, preventing conclusions about causation. There is a need for intervention studies that assess the impact of differing levels of carbohydrate intake in participants with anxiety disorders.

With respect to mechanism, there is evidence that healthy blood sugar regulation is an important factor in mental wellbeing [79]. This relationship may explain the associations seen in the present review between factors that improve blood sugar regulation and lower levels of anxiety symptoms. These include lower intake of sugar and refined carbohydrates, higher fiber intake, regular meals, and caloric restriction.

4.3. Protein

The evidence related to the role of protein in anxiety symptoms is preliminary. There is some evidence suggesting that adequate dietary protein and, in particular, adequate tryptophan, may be important in improving anxiety symptoms. Amino acids serve as the building blocks for neurotransmitter synthesis, with tryptophan needed for the production of serotonin [80]. The established role of serotonin in the pathogenesis of anxiety disorders [81] may explain the potential harm associated with inadequate dietary protein and tryptophan. This evidence is strengthened by the involvement of many participants with diagnosed anxiety disorders in the intervention studies included in the present review. The human experimental studies used doses of tryptophan ranging from 250 mg per day from a food source (squash seeds) to 3 g per day as a supplement. Although these doses are considered to be below the level associated with side-effects [82], the trial that administered 3 g per day reported side effects such as itching, nausea and urinary changes [83]. Tryptophan supplements should not be used in combination with serotonergic medications such as SSRI/SNRI due to the possible risk of precipitating serotonin syndrome [84]. Food sources of tryptophan include egg, soy, seeds, fish and meat [85].

4.4. Fats

Overall, there is significant animal and human evidence that adequate or supplemental omega-3 fatty acids may have anti-anxiety effects. There is early evidence, predominantly from animal studies, that diets high in total fat, cholesterol, or trans fat may have an anxiogenic effect. With respect to a possible mechanism, there is evidence that inflammation plays an important role in the pathogenesis of psychiatric disorders [86], including anxiety [87], and that dietary fats can influence levels of inflammation [88]. Through their effects on enzyme pathways involved in the production of anti-inflammatory cytokines, omega-3 fatty acids contribute to lower levels of inflammation [89]. Conversely, omega-6 fatty acids increase levels of inflammation through increased pro-inflammatory cytokine production. Additionally, there is evidence that omega-3 fatty acids impact oxidative stress [90], neurotransmission [91], and neuroplasticity [92], which are known or hypothesized mechanisms for their use in the treatment of anxiety disorders [93,94]. Dietary omega-3 sources include fish and seafood, as well as flax seeds, chia and hemp seeds.

One somewhat inconsistent finding that has been observed in the present review is the impact of high fat diets. A large number of animal studies (39 of 63) reported a worsening of anxiety symptoms in response to intake of a high-fat diet. In contrast, the studies assessing the ketogenic diet, a diet that is very low in carbohydrates and generally high in fat content, suggest a possible therapeutic benefit. While these findings may be considered conflicting, it is speculated that the type of dietary fats used may have differed, with the high-fat diet delivered to the animals being composed of more omega-6, saturated and trans fatty acids. As such, the type of dietary fat, may be a significant factor in addition to the quantity of fat consumed.

4.5. Vitamins and Minerals

There is significant animal data suggesting an anxiolytic effect of several vitamins and minerals as well as supplemental formulas which deliver a combination or broad range of micronutrients. Given the presence of micronutrients in whole, unprocessed foods such as vegetables, fruit, and whole grains, these findings add evidence to the importance of eating a healthy diet containing a variety of unprocessed foods. Intake of foods that provide a rich source of zinc (oysters, crustaceans, meat, organ meat, leafy and root vegetables [95]), and selenium (Brazil nuts, seafood, meat, beans, and lentils [85]) could be prioritized.

Micronutrients such as zinc and selenium are necessary as coenzymes in the synthesis and regulation of neurotransmitters and neurotrophic factors [96] which may explain their importance in maintaining mental wellbeing. Additionally, B vitamins and folic acid contribute to the methylation balance which is hypothesized to be relevant to the pathophysiology of psychiatric illnesses [97].

4.6. Vegetables, Fruits, and Phytochemicals

There is fairly consistent evidence that vegetables, fruit, and plant constituents may exert anti-anxiety actions; however, the majority of the evidence comes from animal studies.

Caffeine on its own or added to energy drinks appears to be associated with increased anxiety. Whole foods containing caffeine such as coffee, teas and cacao may have beneficial or equivocal impacts on anxiety, likely due to the co-occurrence of caffeine with other beneficial phytochemicals. Vegetables and fruit contribute to lower levels of inflammation and oxidative stress through their phytochemical and antioxidant constituents [98].

4.7. Food Allergy and Intolerance

The body of evidence related to the connection between food allergies and anxiety symptoms is limited and the majority of the evidence pertains to the presence of elevated anxiety symptoms among individuals with celiac disease and the anti-anxiety effects of implementing a gluten-free diet in this population. The presence of neuropsychiatric symptoms in celiac disease is established, with hypothesized mechanisms including micronutrient deficiency due to malabsorption and hyperhomocysteinemia [99]; however, it is unclear how the findings of these studies may apply to anxious individuals unaffected by celiac disease.

4.8. Gut Microbiome

Preliminary evidence suggests that the intake of beneficial microorganisms and prebiotic fiber may be beneficial in the treatment of anxiety. Habitual diet strongly influences the composition of the gut microbiome, thus adding more rationale for the inclusion of fruits, vegetables, fiber, and fermented foods in the diet [100]. Potential mechanisms for the impact of the microbiome on psychiatric wellbeing include the modulation of the production of gut peptides involved in the gut-brain axis [101] and neurotransmitter synthesis [102].

4.9. Strengths and Limitations

Strengths of the present review include an extremely rigorous search strategy intended to capture the full range of publications presenting data on this topic. A priori inclusion criteria and duplicate screening decreased the risk of bias. Completion of the project by an interdisciplinary team including clinicians and researchers contributed a range of perspectives and expertise.

The very large scope of this review was both a strength and limitation. Due to the very large volume of articles included in the review, in-depth analysis of individual articles was not possible. The results of the review may include over-simplification of the findings and a lack of attention to evaluating study quality, assessing study or publication bias, or providing contextual information (e.g., dose). In our data extraction and analysis we did not evaluate of the methods used for assessing participant anxiety symptoms or disorders, Anxiety symptoms can be assessed through a variety of methods including clinician- or self-administered questionnaires, or interviews which may utilize a range of diagnostic criteria. These different methods differ in their reliability as well as the exact nature of the symptoms or disorders that they assess. As a result, the studies included in this review report on relationships between food and a heterogeneous group of outcomes including the presence or absence of different anxiety disorders and a range of anxiety symptoms. The decision to include this heterogenous collection of research was an effort to capture a broad range of data related to this topic.

Another limitation of the present review is the unclear relevance of experimental studies which assessed the impact of high dose supplements of a dietary constituent. Doses of some of the nutrients delivered in trials as dietary supplement, such as zinc and omega-3 fatty acids, can be achieved through dietary modification; however, some of the nutrients, such as vitamin B6 (50 mg/day) were delivered in doses that cannot be achieved with food alone.

Another limitation was the exclusion of studies that failed to report changes in anxiety separately from other outcomes. Several studies that were not included in the present analysis reported 'psychological distress' as a composite of anxiety and depression symptoms but did not report anxiety results alone [103,104]. These studies were excluded from the present analysis as the purpose of this project was to identify research reporting anxiety outcomes specifically; however, it is noted that this resulted in the exclusion of a number of articles ($n = 22$).

The ability to draw conclusions from the data is also limited by a number of factors related to the methodology used in the included studies. This scoping review included a large number of animal studies which may have unclear applicability to humans. There are well established tests designed to measure changes in anxiety levels in animals through monitoring their behavior in a variety of experimental settings [105]; however, the applicability of these results to the human experience of anxiety is inherently limited. The benefits of animal research include the ability to manipulate dietary factors in a highly controlled environment, the ability to observe effects rapidly as a result of the animals' reduced lifespan and the ability to withhold potentially beneficial nutrients. There were also a large number of observational studies, mostly cross-sectional in nature. This type of study cannot draw conclusions about causality. The association between diet and mental health is known to be highly complex and bidirectional. While there is robust evidence that dietary patterns impact the likelihood of developing mental illness [14], there is also evidence that mental illness impacts eating behaviors [106]. This occurs through changes in motivation and appetite that can results from mental illness [107] and metabolic changes, increased appetite and cravings, and gastrointestinal distress [108] that can occur as a results of psychiatric medications [109]. Additionally, confounding factors such as eating disorders may be responsible for associations that are present. Given this bidirectional relationship, the findings of cross-sectional studies have limited ability to answer the question of how food impacts anxiety. While a small number of prospective observational studies were identified in the present review, additional prospective studies are needed in order to accurately assess the impact of dietary patterns on the development of mental disorders, particularly the avoidance of potentially beneficial foods and increased intake of potentially harmful foods, which cannot be studied using an experimental design for ethical reasons.

Another important consideration when interpreting the study findings is the potential for difference between short- and long-term impacts of food on anxiety symptoms. As previously mentioned, it is known that the relationship between mental health symptoms and diet choices is bidirectional; emotional symptoms may drive eating behavior because of their immediate effects on the mitigation of emotional symptoms. The term "comfort eating" has been used to describe the phenomenon where individuals consume foods, especially those higher in calories, sugar, and fat, in response to negative affect [110]. Evidence from mechanistic studies suggest that corticosterone, a stress hormone, positively influences an animal's intake of a sweet beverage [111] and that consumption of comfort food decreases mRNA production of hormones related to the stress response in animals [110]. It has been hypothesized that comfort eating is a behavior that decreases the stress-response during the experience of anxiety [110]. This phenomenon might explain some of the mixed finding of the present study. When considering the studies using "unhealthy", "cafeteria", or Western diets in animal models, 17 studies reported a decrease in anxiety symptoms and 21 reported an increase in anxiety symptoms. In contrast, of the 17 human observational studies assessing the relationship between unhealthy diet patterns and anxiety symptoms, 15 reported an association with more anxiety, and two reported no association. The mixed findings among the animal studies may be due to the duration of the experiment. Many of these studies assessed the impact of three to four weeks of the diet exposure on animal behavior and many of the studies reporting benefit assessed the impact of the diet on animals experiencing stress. The reported beneficial effects may be capturing the short-term stress-reducing effect of foods high in sugar and fat. In contrast, the human observational studies may have been capturing the effects of chronic consumption of unhealthy diets.

Another limitation that impacts the ability to draw clear conclusions from the present data is the enormous complexity of studying nutritional science. When considering the role of macronutrients (carbohydrates, protein, and fat), it is necessary to consider both the amount and type of the nutrient consumed. As highlighted previously, studies which categorized dietary patterns as high or low in macronutrients such as fat or carbohydrates may not have considered the types of fat or carbohydrates being consumed. Given the highly different health impacts of complex and refined carbohydrates, significant attention should be given to the studies differentiating these rather than those assessing total carbohydrates only.

Only a small number of intervention studies involved participants with anxiety disorders, many involved healthy participants or individuals with medical illnesses such as irritable bowel syndrome, diabetes, and cardiovascular disease. This has several implications. First, many of these studies were designed to assess cardiometabolic outcomes primarily and the studies may have not been adequately powered to detect changes in mental health symptoms. Secondly, the participants recruited to participate in these studies related to physical illness may have had low baseline levels of anxiety symptoms making it difficult to detect statistically significant changes in symptoms or becoming more susceptible to other scale attenuation effects (e.g., floor and ceiling effects). Thirdly, the impact of a nutritional intervention on a healthy or non-anxious individual may not be relevant to understanding how the intervention might impact individuals with clinically significant anxiety disorders. There is a clear need for intervention studies enrolling participants with anxiety disorders or elevated anxiety symptoms. Similarly, studies designed with changes in mental health symptoms as the primary outcomes are needed.

5. Conclusions

Although the results of this review reflect a field of study that is preliminary and emerging, the findings are consistent with established evidence about healthy eating patterns [112]. There is evidence of an association between healthy eating patterns and reduced anxiety symptoms. In the absence of a contraindication such as an allergy or specific medical condition, dietary interventions are considered low in risk, cost-effective [113], may confer secondary benefit to physical aspects of health and have at least some evidence suggesting a beneficial effect. However, the delivery of nutritional counselling as part of the treatment of anxiety disorders by primary care, psychiatry, dieticians, naturopaths, or other care providers is currently limited.

Prospective observational studies are needed to more clearly establish the causal role of diet factors in the development and progression of anxiety disorders. High quality intervention studies involving participants with anxiety disorders are warranted in order to evaluate the therapeutic potential of nutrition interventions in the management of anxiety disorders.

Supplementary Materials: The following are available online at https://www.mdpi.com/article/10.3390/nu13124418/s1, File S1: Search Strategy, File S2: Excluded studies, File S3: All included studies.

Author Contributions: Conceptualization, M.A., L.L. and K.C.; methodology, M.A., L.L. and K.C.; data extraction, M.A., D.R., T.S., N.S., V.C., T.R. and I.C. formal analysis, M.A. and L.L.; writing—original draft preparation, M.A.; writing—review and editing, L.L., U.N., D.R., T.S., N.S., V.C., T.R., I.C. and K.C. All authors have read and agreed to the published version of the manuscript.

Funding: This research received no external funding.

Institutional Review Board Statement: Not applicable.

Informed Consent Statement: Not applicable.

Data Availability Statement: Supporting data available on request.

Acknowledgments: Becky Skidmore: design of search strategy.

Conflicts of Interest: The authors declare no conflict of interest.

References

1. Gale, C.K.; Millichamp, J. Generalised anxiety disorder. *BMJ Clin. Evid.* **2011**, *2011*, 1002.
2. Kim, Y.-K. Panic Disorder: Current Research and Management Approaches. *Psychiatry Investig.* **2019**, *16*, 1–3. [CrossRef] [PubMed]
3. Wittchen, H.-U.; Gloster, A.T.; Beesdo-Baum, K.; Fava, G.A.; Craske, M.G. Agoraphobia: A review of the diagnostic classificatory position and criteria. *Depress. Anxiety* **2010**, *27*, 113–133. [CrossRef] [PubMed]
4. Glue, P.; Canton, J.; Scott, K.M. Optimal treatment of social phobia: Systematic review and meta-analysis. *Neuropsychiatr. Dis. Treat.* **2012**, *8*, 203–215. [CrossRef]
5. Eaton, W.W.; Bienvenu, O.J.; Miloyan, B. Specific phobias. *Lancet Psychiatry* **2018**, *5*, 678–686. [CrossRef]
6. Louise, P.; Siobhan, O.; Louise, M.; Jean, G.; Pelletier, L.; O'Donnell, S.; McRae, L.; Grenier, J. The burden of generalized anxiety disorder in Canada. *Health Promot. Chronic Dis. Prev. Can.* **2017**, *37*, 54–62. [CrossRef]
7. Saarni, S.I.; Suvisaari, J.; Sintonen, H.; Pirkola, S.; Koskinen, S.; Aromaa, A.; Lönnqvist, J. Impact of psychiatric disorders on health-related quality of life: General population survey. *Br. J. Psychiatry* **2007**, *190*, 326–332. [CrossRef]
8. Revicki, D.A.; Travers, K.; Wyrwich, K.W.; Svedsäter, H.; Locklear, J.; Mattera, M.S.; Sheehan, D.V.; Montgomery, S. Humanistic and economic burden of generalized anxiety disorder in North America and Europe. *J. Affect. Disord.* **2012**, *140*, 103–112. [CrossRef]
9. Kessler, R.C.; McGonagle, K.A.; Zhao, S.; Nelson, C.B.; Hughes, M.; Eshleman, S.; Wittchen, H.-U.; Kendler, K.S. Lifetime and 12-Month Prevalence of DSM-III-R Psychiatric Disorders in the United States. *Arch. Gen. Psychiatry* **1994**, *51*, 8–19. [CrossRef]
10. Gliatto, M.F. Generalized anxiety disorder. *Am. Fam. Physician* **2000**, *62*, 1591–1600.
11. Collins, K.A.; Westra, H.A.; Dozois, D.J.; Burns, D.D. Gaps in accessing treatment for anxiety and depression: Challenges for the delivery of care. *Clin. Psychol. Rev.* **2004**, *24*, 583–616. [CrossRef] [PubMed]
12. Jacka, F.N.; O'Neil, A.; Opie, R.; Itsiopoulos, C.; Cotton, S.; Mohebbi, M.; Castle, D.; Dash, S.; Mihalopoulos, C.; Chatterton, M.L.; et al. A randomised controlled trial of dietary improvement for adults with major depression (the 'SMILES' trial). *BMC Med.* **2017**, *15*, 23. [CrossRef]
13. Parletta, N.; Zarnowiecki, D.; Cho, J.; Wilson, A.; Bogomolova, S.; Villani, A.; Itsiopoulos, C.; Niyonsenga, T.; Blunden, S.; Meyer, B.; et al. A Mediterranean-style dietary intervention supplemented with fish oil improves diet quality and mental health in people with depression: A randomized controlled trial (HELFIMED). *Nutr. Neurosci.* **2019**, *22*, 474–487. [CrossRef]
14. Marx, W.; Moseley, G.; Berk, M.; Jacka, F. Nutritional psychiatry: The present state of the evidence. *Proc. Nutr. Soc.* **2017**, *76*, 427–436. [CrossRef] [PubMed]
15. Xu, Y.; Zeng, L.; Zou, K.; Shan, S.; Wang, X.; Xiong, J.; Zhao, L.; Zhang, L.; Cheng, G. Role of dietary factors in the prevention and treatment for depression: An umbrella review of meta-analyses of prospective studies. *Transl. Psychiatry* **2021**, *11*, 478. [CrossRef]
16. Arksey, H.; O'Malley, L. Scoping studies: Towards a methodological framework. *Int. J. Soc. Res. Methodol.* **2005**, *8*, 19–32. [CrossRef]
17. Aucoin, M.; LaChance, L.; Cooley, K.; Kidd, S. Diet and Psychosis: A Scoping Review. *Neuropsychobiology* **2020**, *79*, 20–42. [CrossRef]
18. Gates, A.; Johnson, C.; Hartling, L. Technology-assisted title and abstract screening for systematic reviews: A retrospective evaluation of the Abstrackr machine learning tool. *Syst. Rev.* **2018**, *7*, 45. [CrossRef]
19. Rathbone, J.; Hoffmann, T.; Glasziou, P. Faster title and abstract screening? Evaluating Abstrackr, a semi-automated online screening program for systematic reviewers. *Syst. Rev.* **2015**, *4*, 80. [CrossRef] [PubMed]
20. Gates, A.; Gates, M.; Sebastianski, M.; Guitard, S.; Elliott, S.A.; Hartling, L. The semi-automation of title and abstract screening: A retrospective exploration of ways to leverage Abstrackr's relevance predictions in systematic and rapid reviews. *BMC Med. Res. Methodol.* **2020**, *20*, 139. [CrossRef]
21. Clappison, E.; Hadjivassiliou, M.; Zis, P. Psychiatric Manifestations of Coeliac Disease, a Systematic Review and Meta-Analysis. *Nutrients* **2020**, *12*, 142. [CrossRef]
22. Hunsche, C.; de Toda, I.M.; De la Fuente, M. Impacts of the late adulthood diet-induced obesity onset on behavior, immune function, redox state and life span of male and female mice. *Brain Behav. Immun.* **2019**, *78*, 65–77. [CrossRef]
23. Souza, C.; Moreira, J.D.; Siqueira, I.; Pereira, A.; Rieger, D.; Souza, D.; Souza, T.; Portela, L.; Perry, M. Highly palatable diet consumption increases protein oxidation in rat frontal cortex and anxiety-like behavior. *Life Sci.* **2007**, *81*, 198–203. [CrossRef]
24. Clemente-Suárez, V.J. Multidisciplinary intervention in the treatment of mixed anxiety and depression disorder. *Physiol. Behav.* **2020**, *219*, 112858. [CrossRef]
25. Null, G.; Pennesi, L.; Feldman, M. Nutrition and Lifestyle Intervention on Mood and Neurological Disorders. *J. Evid.-Based Integr. Med.* **2017**, *22*, 68–74. [CrossRef]
26. Cooley, K.; Szczurko, O.; Perri, D.; Mills, E.J.; Bernhardt, B.; Zhou, Q.; Seely, D. Naturopathic Care for Anxiety: A Randomized Controlled Trial ISRCTN78958974. *PLoS ONE* **2009**, *4*, e6628. [CrossRef]
27. Forsyth, A.; Deane, F.P.; Williams, P. A lifestyle intervention for primary care patients with depression and anxiety: A randomised controlled trial. *Psychiatry Res.* **2015**, *230*, 537–544. [CrossRef]
28. Laporte, D.J. Treatment response in obese binge eaters: Preliminary results using a very low calorie diet (VLCD) and behavior therapy. *Addict. Behav.* **1992**, *17*, 247–257. [CrossRef]

29. Ein, N.; Armstrong, B.; Vickers, K. The effect of a very low calorie diet on subjective depressive symptoms and anxiety: Meta-analysis and systematic review. *Int. J. Obes.* **2018**, *43*, 1444–1455. [CrossRef]
30. Jebeile, H.; Gow, M.L.; Baur, L.A.; Garnett, S.P.; Paxton, S.J.; Lister, N.B. Association of Pediatric Obesity Treatment, Including a Dietary Component, with Change in Depression and Anxiety: A Systematic Review and Meta-analysis. *JAMA Pediatr.* **2019**, *173*, e192841. [CrossRef] [PubMed]
31. Hillman, L.C.; Stace, N.H.; Pomare, E.W. Irritable bowel patients and their long-term response to a high fiber diet. *Am. J. Gastroenterol.* **1984**, *79*, 1–7.
32. Christensen, L.; Krietsch, K.; White, B.; Stagner, B. Impact of a dietary change on emotional distress. *J. Abnorm. Psychol.* **1985**, *94*, 565–579. [CrossRef]
33. Mohammed, H.; Ghosh, S.; Vuvor, F.; Mensah-Armah, S.; Steiner-Asiedu, M. Dietary intake and the dynamics of stress, hypertension and obesity in a peri-urban community in Accra. *Ghana Med. J.* **2016**, *50*, 16–21. [CrossRef] [PubMed]
34. Mesgarani, M.; Hosseinbor, M.; Shafiee, S.; Sarkoubi, R. The Relationship of Parental Mental Health and Dietary Pattern with Adolescent Mental Health. *Int. J. High Risk Behav. Addict.* **2016**, *5*, e26616. [CrossRef] [PubMed]
35. Hudson, C.; Hudson, S.; MacKenzie, J. Protein-source tryptophan as an efficacious treatment for social anxiety disorder: A pilot studyThis article is one of a selection of papers published in this special issue (part 1 of 2) on the Safety and Efficacy of Natural Health Products. *Can. J. Physiol. Pharmacol.* **2007**, *85*, 928–932. [CrossRef] [PubMed]
36. Capello, A.E.; Markus, C.R. Effect of sub chronic tryptophan supplementation on stress-induced cortisol and appetite in subjects differing in 5-HTTLPR genotype and trait neuroticism. *Psychoneuroendocrinology* **2014**, *45*, 96–107. [CrossRef] [PubMed]
37. Smith, C.A.; Shewamene, Z.; Galbally, M.; Schmied, V.; Dahlen, H. The effect of complementary medicines and therapies on maternal anxiety and depression in pregnancy: A systematic review and meta-analysis. *J. Affect. Disord.* **2019**, *245*, 428–439. [CrossRef]
38. Deane, K.H.O.; Jimoh, O.F.; Biswas, P.; O'Brien, A.; Hanson, S.; Abdelhamid, A.S.; Fox, C.; Hooper, L. Omega-3 and polyunsaturated fat for prevention of depression and anxiety symptoms: Systematic review and meta-analysis of randomised trials. *Br. J. Psychiatry* **2021**, *218*, 135–142. [CrossRef]
39. Su, K.-P.; Tseng, P.-T.; Lin, P.-Y.; Okubo, R.; Chen, T.-Y.; Chen, Y.-W.; Matsuoka, Y.J. Association of Use of Omega-3 Polyunsaturated Fatty Acids with Changes in Severity of Anxiety Symptoms: A Systematic Review and Meta-analysis. *JAMA Netw. Open* **2018**, *1*, e182327. [CrossRef]
40. Yehuda, S.; Rabinovitz, S.; Mostofsky, D.I. Mixture of essential fatty acids lowers test anxiety. *Nutr. Neurosci.* **2005**, *8*, 265–267. [CrossRef] [PubMed]
41. Abdul-Razzak, K.K.; Almanasrah, S.O.; Obeidat, B.A.; Khasawneh, A.G. Vitamin D is a potential antidepressant in psychiatric outpatients. *Int. J. Clin. Pharmacol. Ther.* **2018**, *56*, 585–596. [CrossRef]
42. Rucklidge, J.J.; Andridge, R.; Gorman, B.; Blampied, N.; Gordon, H.; Boggis, A. Shaken but unstirred? Effects of micronutrients on stress and trauma after an earthquake: RCT evidence comparing formulas and doses. *Hum. Psychopharmacol. Clin. Exp.* **2012**, *27*, 440–454. [CrossRef] [PubMed]
43. Gautam, M.; Agrawal, M.; Gautam, M.; Sharma, P.; Gautam, A.S.; Gautam, S. Role of antioxidants in generalised anxiety disorder and depression. *Indian J. Psychiatry* **2012**, *54*, 244–247. [CrossRef]
44. Jaatinen, N.; Korpela, R.; Poussa, T.; Turpeinen, A.; Mustonen, S.; Merilahti, J.; Peuhkuri, K. Effects of daily intake of yoghurt enriched with bioactive components on chronic stress responses: A double-blinded randomized controlled trial. *Int. J. Food Sci. Nutr.* **2013**, *65*, 507–514. [CrossRef] [PubMed]
45. Russo, A. Decreased Zinc and Increased Copper in Individuals with Anxiety. *Nutr. Metab. Insights* **2011**, *4*, NMI.S6349. [CrossRef]
46. Choi, E.B.; Lee, J.E.; Hwang, J.-Y. Fruit and vegetable intakes in relation to behavioral outcomes associated with a nutrition education intervention in preschoolers. *Nutr. Res. Pract.* **2018**, *12*, 521–526. [CrossRef] [PubMed]
47. Conner, T.S.; Brookie, K.L.; Carr, A.C.; Mainvil, L.A.; Vissers, M.C.M. Let them eat fruit! The effect of fruit and vegetable consumption on psychological well-being in young adults: A randomized controlled trial. *PLoS ONE* **2017**, *12*, e0171206. [CrossRef]
48. Smith, A.P.; Rogers, R. Positive Effects of a Healthy Snack (Fruit) Versus an Unhealthy Snack (Chocolate/Crisps) on Subjective Reports of Mental and Physical Health: A Preliminary Intervention Study. *Front. Nutr.* **2014**, *1*, 10. [CrossRef]
49. Camfield, D.; Stough, C.; Farrimond, J.; Scholey, A.B. Acute effects of tea constituents L-theanine, caffeine, and epigallocatechin gallate on cognitive function and mood: A systematic review and meta-analysis. *Nutr. Rev.* **2014**, *72*, 507–522. [CrossRef]
50. Hieu, T.H.; Dibas, M.; Dila, K.A.S.; Sherif, N.A.; Hashmi, M.U.; Mahmoud, M.; Trang, N.T.T.; Abdullah, L.; Nghia, T.L.B.; Mai Nhu, Y.; et al. Therapeutic efficacy and safety of chamomile for state anxiety, generalized anxiety disorder, insomnia, and sleep quality: A systematic review and meta-analysis of randomized trials and quasi-randomized trials. *Phytotherapy Res.* **2019**, *33*, 1604–1615. [CrossRef]
51. Marx, W.; Lane, M.; Rocks, T.; Ruusunen, A.; Loughman, A.; Lopresti, A.; Marshall, S.; Berk, M.; Jacka, F.; Dean, O.M. Effect of saffron supplementation on symptoms of depression and anxiety: A systematic review and meta-analysis. *Nutr. Rev.* **2019**, *77*, 557–571. [CrossRef]
52. Fusar-Poli, L.; Vozza, L.; Gabbiadini, A.; Vanella, A.; Concas, I.; Tinacci, S.; Petralia, A.; Signorelli, M.; Aguglia, E. Curcumin for depression: A meta-analysis. *Crit. Rev. Food Sci. Nutr.* **2020**, *60*, 2643–2653. [CrossRef] [PubMed]

53. Ng, Q.X.; Koh, S.S.H.; Chan, H.W.; Ho, C.Y.X. Clinical Use of Curcumin in Depression: A Meta-Analysis. *J. Am. Med. Dir. Assoc.* **2017**, *18*, 503–508. [CrossRef]
54. Farzaei, M.H.; Rahimi, R.; Nikfar, S.; Abdollahi, M. Effect of resveratrol on cognitive and memory performance and mood: A meta-analysis of 225 patients. *Pharmacol. Res.* **2018**, *128*, 338–344. [CrossRef]
55. Keefe, J.R.; Guo, W.; Li, Q.S.; Amsterdam, J.D.; Mao, J.J. An exploratory study of salivary cortisol changes during chamomile extract therapy of moderate to severe generalized anxiety disorder. *J. Psychiatr. Res.* **2018**, *96*, 189–195. [CrossRef] [PubMed]
56. Amsterdam, J.D.; Li, Y.; Soeller, I.; Rockwell, K.; Mao, J.J.; Shults, J. A Randomized, Double-Blind, Placebo-Controlled Trial of Oral Matricaria recutita (Chamomile) Extract Therapy for Generalized Anxiety Disorder. *J. Clin. Psychopharmacol.* **2009**, *29*, 378–382. [CrossRef]
57. Mao, J.J.; Xie, S.X.; Keefe, J.R.; Soeller, I.; Li, Q.S.; Amsterdam, J.D. Long-term chamomile (*Matricaria chamomilla* L.) treatment for generalized anxiety disorder: A randomized clinical trial. *Phytomedicine* **2016**, *23*, 1735–1742. [CrossRef]
58. Jafarnia, N.; Ghorbani, Z.; Nokhostin, M.; Manayi, A.; Nourimajd, S.; Jahromi, S.R. Effect of Saffron (*Crocus satious* L.) as an Add-On Therapy to Sertraline in Mild to Moderate Generalized Anxiety Disorder: A Double Blind Randomized Controlled Trial. *Arch. Neurosci.* **2017**, *4*, e14332. [CrossRef]
59. Milajerdi, A.; Jazayeri, S.; Shirzadi, E.; Hashemzadeh, N.; Azizgol, A.; Djazayery, A.; Esmaillzadeh, A.; Akhondzadeh, S. The effects of alcoholic extract of saffron (*Crocus satious* L.) on mild to moderate comorbid depression-anxiety, sleep quality, and life satisfaction in type 2 diabetes mellitus: A double-blind, randomized and placebo-controlled clinical trial. *Complement. Ther. Med.* **2018**, *41*, 196–202. [CrossRef]
60. Sudheeran, S.P.; Jacob, D.; Mulakal, J.N.; Nair, G.G.; Maliakel, A.; Maliakel, B.; Ramadasan, K.; Krishnakumar, I.M. Safety, Tolerance, and Enhanced Efficacy of a Bioavailable Formulation of Curcumin with Fenugreek Dietary Fiber on Occupational Stress: A Randomized, Double-Blind, Placebo-Controlled Pilot Study. *J. Clin. Psychopharmacol.* **2016**, *36*, 236–243. [CrossRef]
61. Sarris, J.; Byrne, G.J.; Cribb, L.; Oliver, G.; Murphy, J.; Macdonald, P.; Nazareth, S.; Karamacoska, D.; Galea, S.; Short, A.; et al. L-theanine in the adjunctive treatment of generalized anxiety disorder: A double-blind, randomised, placebo-controlled trial. *J. Psychiatr. Res.* **2019**, *110*, 31–37. [CrossRef]
62. Pinto-Sanchez, M.I.; Hall, G.B.; Ghajar, K.; Nardelli, A.; Bolino, C.; Lau, J.T.; Martin, F.-P.; Cominetti, O.; Welsh, C.; Rieder, A.; et al. Probiotic Bifidobacterium longum NCC3001 Reduces Depression Scores and Alters Brain Activity: A Pilot Study in Patients with Irritable Bowel Syndrome. *Gastroenterology* **2017**, *153*, 448–459.e8. [CrossRef]
63. Eskandarzadeh, S.; Effatpanah, M.; Khosravi-Darani, K.; Askari, R.; Hosseini, A.F.; Reisian, M.; Jazayeri, S. Efficacy of a multispecies probiotic as adjunctive therapy in generalized anxiety disorder: A double blind, randomized, placebo-controlled trial. *Nutr. Neurosci.* **2021**, *24*, 102–108. [CrossRef] [PubMed]
64. Liu, B.; He, Y.; Wang, M.; Liu, J.; Ju, Y.; Zhang, Y.; Liu, T.; Li, L.; Li, Q. Efficacy of probiotics on anxiety-A meta-analysis of randomized controlled trials. *Depress. Anxiety* **2018**, *35*, 935–945. [CrossRef] [PubMed]
65. Liu, R.T.; Walsh, R.F.L.; Sheehan, A.E. Prebiotics and probiotics for depression and anxiety: A systematic review and meta-analysis of controlled clinical trials. *Neurosci. Biobehav. Rev.* **2019**, *102*, 13–23. [CrossRef]
66. Reis, D.J.; Ilardi, S.S.; Punt, S.E.W. The anxiolytic effect of probiotics: A systematic review and meta-analysis of the clinical and preclinical literature. *PLoS ONE* **2018**, *13*, e0199041. [CrossRef]
67. Del Olmo, N.; Blanco-Gandia, M.C.; Mateos-Garcia, A.; Del Rio, D.; Minarro, J.; Ruiz-Gayo, M.; Rodríguez-Arias, M. Differential Impact of Ad Libitum or Intermittent High-Fat Diets on Bingeing Ethanol-Mediated Behaviors. *Nutrients* **2019**, *11*, 2253. [CrossRef]
68. Dornellas, A.P.S.; Boldarine, V.T.; Pedroso, A.P.; Carvalho, L.O.T.; de Andrade, I.S.; Vulcani-Freitas, T.M.; dos Santos, C.C.C.; da Penha Oller do Nascimento, C.M.; Oyama, L.M.; Ribeiro, E.B. High-Fat Feeding Improves Anxiety-Type Behavior Induced by Ovariectomy in Rats. *Front. Neurosci.* **2018**, *12*, 557. [CrossRef] [PubMed]
69. Segat, H.; Barcelos, R.; Metz, V.; Rosa, H.; Roversi, K.; Antoniazzi, C.; Vey, L.; Kronbauer, M.; Veit, J.; Piccolo, J.; et al. Influence of physical activity on addiction parameters of rats exposed to amphetamine which were previously supplemented with hydrogenated vegetable fat. *Brain Res. Bull.* **2017**, *135*, 69–76. [CrossRef] [PubMed]
70. Segev, Y.; Livne, A.; Mints, M.; Rosenblum, K. Concurrence of High Fat Diet and APOE Gene Induces Allele Specific Metabolic and Mental Stress Changes in a Mouse Model of Alzheimer's Disease. *Front. Behav. Neurosci.* **2016**, *10*, 170. [CrossRef]
71. Otsuka, A.; Shiuchi, T.; Chikahisa, S.; Shimizu, N.; Séi, H. Sufficient intake of high-fat food attenuates stress-induced social avoidance behavior. *Life Sci.* **2019**, *219*, 219–230. [CrossRef]
72. Haleem, D.J.; Mahmood, K. Brain serotonin in high-fat diet-induced weight gain, anxiety and spatial memory in rats. *Nutr. Neurosci.* **2021**, *24*, 226–235. [CrossRef] [PubMed]
73. Hu, F.B.; Manson, J.E.; Willett, W.C. Types of Dietary Fat and Risk of Coronary Heart Disease: A Critical Review. *J. Am. Coll. Nutr.* **2001**, *20*, 5–19. [CrossRef] [PubMed]
74. Ramsden, C.E.; Zamora, D.; Majchrzak-Hong, S.; Faurot, K.; Broste, S.K.; Frantz, R.; Davis, J.M.; Ringel, A.; Suchindran, C.M.; Hibbeln, J.R. Re-evaluation of the traditional diet-heart hypothesis: Analysis of recovered data from Minnesota Coronary Experiment (1968–73). *BMJ* **2016**, *353*, i1246. [CrossRef] [PubMed]
75. Sergentanis, T.; Chelmi, M.-E.; Liampas, A.; Yfanti, C.-M.; Panagouli, E.; Vlachopapadopoulou, E.; Michalacos, S.; Bacopoulou, F.; Psaltopoulou, T.; Tsitsika, A. Vegetarian Diets and Eating Disorders in Adolescents and Young Adults: A Systematic Review. *Children* **2020**, *8*, 12. [CrossRef]

76. Swinbourne, J.M.; Touyz, S. The co-morbidity of eating disorders and anxiety disorders: A review. *Eur. Eat. Disord. Rev.* **2007**, *15*, 253–274. [CrossRef]
77. Woo, K.S.; Kwok, T.C.; Celermajer, D.S. Vegan Diet, Subnormal Vitamin B-12 Status and Cardiovascular Health. *Nutrients* **2014**, *6*, 3259–3273. [CrossRef]
78. Lakin, V.; Haggarty, P.; Abramovich, D.; Ashton, J.; Moffat, C.; McNeill, G.; Danielian, P.; Grubb, D. Dietary intake and tissue concentration of fatty acids in omnivore, vegetarian and diabetic pregnancy. *Prostaglandins Leukot. Essent. Fat. Acids* **1998**, *59*, 209–220. [CrossRef]
79. Anderson, R.J.; Grigsby, A.B.; Freedland, K.E.; De Groot, M.; McGill, J.B.; Clouse, R.E.; Lustman, P.J. Anxiety and poor glycemic control: A meta-analytic review of the literature. *Int. J. Psychiatry Med.* **2002**, *32*, 235–247. [CrossRef]
80. Moja, E.A.; Cipolla, P.; Castoldi, D.; Tofanetti, O. Dose-response decrease in plasma tryptophan and in brain tryptophan and serotonin after tryptophan-free amino acid mixtures in rats. *Life Sci.* **1989**, *44*, 971–976. [CrossRef]
81. Stein, D.J.; Stahl, S. Serotonin and anxiety: Current models. *Int. Clin. Psychopharmacol.* **2000**, *15*, S1–S6. [CrossRef] [PubMed]
82. Cynober, L.; Bier, D.M.; Kadowaki, M.; Morris, J.S.M.; Elango, R.; Smriga, M. Proposals for Upper Limits of Safe Intake for Arginine and Tryptophan in Young Adults and an Upper Limit of Safe Intake for Leucine in the Elderly. *J. Nutr.* **2016**, *146*, 2652S–2654S. [CrossRef] [PubMed]
83. Seltzer, S.; Dewart, D.; Pollack, R.L.; Jackson, E. The effects of dietary tryptophan on chronic maxillofacial pain and experimental pain tolerance. *J. Psychiatr. Res.* **1982**, *17*, 181–186. [CrossRef]
84. Alusik, S.; Kalatova, D.; Paluch, Z. Serotonin syndrome. *Neuroendocrinol. Lett.* **2014**, *35*, 265–273.
85. U.S. Department of Agriculture, Agricultural Research Service. FoodData Central. 2019. Available online: Fdc.nal.usda.gov (accessed on 22 September 2021).
86. Firth, J.; Veronese, N.; Cotter, J.; Shivappa, N.; Hebert, J.R.; Ee, C.; Smith, L.; Stubbs, B.; Jackson, S.E.; Sarris, J. What Is the Role of Dietary Inflammation in Severe Mental Illness? A Review of Observational and Experimental Findings. *Front. Psychiatry* **2019**, *10*, 350. [CrossRef] [PubMed]
87. Salim, S.; Chugh, G.; Asghar, M. Inflammation in Anxiety. *Adv. Protein Chem. Struct. Biol.* **2012**, *88*, 1–25. [CrossRef]
88. Calder, P.C. Polyunsaturated fatty acids and inflammation. *Prostaglandins Leukot. Essent. Fat. Acids* **2006**, *75*, 197–202. [CrossRef]
89. Bäck, M.; Hansson, G.K. Omega-3 fatty acids, cardiovascular risk, and the resolution of inflammation. *FASEB J.* **2019**, *33*, 1536–1539. [CrossRef]
90. Chen, J.; Wang, D.; Zong, Y.; Yang, X. DHA Protects Hepatocytes from Oxidative Injury through GPR120/ERK-Mediated Mitophagy. *Int. J. Mol. Sci.* **2021**, *22*, 5675. [CrossRef]
91. DeLion, S.; Chalon, S.; Hérault, J.; Guilloteau, D.; Besnard, J.C.; Durand, G. Chronic dietary alpha-linolenic acid deficiency alters dopaminergic and serotoninergic neurotransmission in rats. *J. Nutr.* **1994**, *124*, 2466–2476. [CrossRef]
92. Marino, A.; Cuzzocrea, S. n-3 Fatty Acids: Role in Neurogenesis and Neuroplasticity. *Curr. Med. Chem.* **2013**, *20*, 2953–2963. [CrossRef]
93. Gałecki, P.; Mossakowska-Wójcik, J.; Talarowska, M. The anti-inflammatory mechanism of antidepressants—SSRIs, SNRIs. *Prog. Neuro-Psychopharmacol. Biol. Psychiatry* **2018**, *80*, 291–294. [CrossRef] [PubMed]
94. Branchi, I.; Santarelli, S.; Capoccia, S.; Poggini, S.; D'Andrea, I.; Cirulli, F.; Alleva, E. Antidepressant Treatment Outcome Depends on the Quality of the Living Environment: A Pre-Clinical Investigation in Mice. *PLoS ONE* **2013**, *8*, e62226. [CrossRef]
95. Solomons, N.W. Dietary Sources of Zinc and Factors Affecting its Bioavailability. *Food Nutr. Bull.* **2001**, *22*, 138–154. [CrossRef]
96. Rucklidge, J.J.; Kaplan, B.J. Broad-spectrum micronutrient formulas for the treatment of psychiatric symptoms: A systematic review. *Expert Rev. Neurother.* **2013**, *13*, 49–73. [CrossRef] [PubMed]
97. Abdolmaleky, H.M.; Smith, C.; Faraone, S.; Shafa, R.; Stone, W.; Glatt, S.; Tsuang, M.T. Methylomics in psychiatry: Modulation of gene-environment interactions may be through DNA methylation. *Am. J. Med. Genet.* **2004**, *127B*, 51–59. [CrossRef] [PubMed]
98. Zhu, F.; Du, B.; Xu, B. Anti-inflammatory effects of phytochemicals from fruits, vegetables, and food legumes: A review. *Crit. Rev. Food Sci. Nutr.* **2018**, *58*, 1260–1270. [CrossRef]
99. Trovato, C.M.; Raucci, U.; Valitutti, F.; Montuori, M.; Villa, M.P.; Cucchiara, S.; Parisi, P. Neuropsychiatric manifestations in celiac disease. *Epilepsy Behav.* **2019**, *99*, 106393. [CrossRef] [PubMed]
100. Wastyk, H.C.; Fragiadakis, G.K.; Perelman, D.; Dahan, D.; Merrill, B.D.; Yu, F.B.; Topf, M.; Gonzalez, C.G.; Van Treuren, W.; Han, S.; et al. Gut-microbiota-targeted diets modulate human immune status. *Cell* **2021**, *184*, 4137–4153.e14. [CrossRef]
101. Lach, G.; Schellekens, H.; Dinan, T.G.; Cryan, J.F. Anxiety, Depression, and the Microbiome: A Role for Gut Peptides. *Neurotherapeutics* **2018**, *15*, 36–59. [CrossRef] [PubMed]
102. Shafiq, J.; Khan, B.; Saleem, F.; Abbas, G.; Ahmed, A. Gut microbiome interferes with host tryptophan metabolism pathway and regulate basal anxiety–like behavior. *Int. J. Infect. Dis.* **2020**, *101*, 5. [CrossRef]
103. Arbour-Nicitopoulos, K.P.; Faulkner, G.; Irving, H.M. Multiple Health-Risk Behaviour and Psychological Distress in Adolescence. *J. Can. Acad. Child Adolesc. Psychiatry* **2012**, *21*, 171–178. [PubMed]
104. Grønning, K.; Espnes, G.A.; Nguyen, C.; Rodrigues, A.M.F.; Gregorio, M.J.; Sousa, R.; Canhão, H.; André, B. Psychological distress in elderly people is associated with diet, wellbeing, health status, social support and physical functioning—A HUNT3 study. *BMC Geriatr.* **2018**, *18*, 205. [CrossRef]
105. Steimer, T. Animal models of anxiety disorders in rats and mice: Some conceptual issues. *Dialog. Clin. Neurosci.* **2011**, *13*, 495–506.

106. van der Pols, J.C. Nutrition and mental health: Bidirectional associations and multidimensional measures. *Public Health Nutr.* **2018**, *21*, 829–830.
107. Macht, M.; Roth, S.; Ellgring, H. Chocolate eating in healthy men during experimentally induced sadness and joy. *Appetite* **2002**, *39*, 147–158. [CrossRef]
108. Willner, P.; Benton, D.; Brown, E.; Cheeta, S.; Roderique-Davies, G.; Morgan, J.; Morgan, M. "Depression" increases "craving" for sweet rewards in animal and human models of depression and craving. *Psychopharmacology* **1998**, *136*, 272–283. [CrossRef]
109. Shobo, M.; Yamada, H.; Mihara, T.; Kondo, Y.; Irie, M.; Harada, K.; Ni, K.; Matsuoka, N.; Kayama, Y. Two models for weight gain and hyperphagia as side effects of atypical antipsychotics in male rats: Validation with olanzapine and ziprasidone. *Behav. Brain Res.* **2011**, *216*, 561–568. [CrossRef]
110. Dallman, M.F.; Pecoraro, N.; Akana, S.F.; la Fleur, S.E.; Gomez, F.; Houshyar, H.; Bell, M.E.; Bhatnagar, S.; Laugero, K.D.; Manalo, S. Chronic stress and obesity: A new view of "comfort food". *Proc. Natl. Acad. Sci. USA* **2003**, *100*, 11696–11701. [CrossRef] [PubMed]
111. Bhatnagar, S.; Bell, M.E.; Liang, J.; Soriano, L.; Nagy, T.R.; Dallman, M.F. Corticosterone Facilitates Saccharin Intake in Adrenalectomized Rats: Does Corticosterone Increase Stimulus Salience? *J. Neuroendocr.* **2000**, *12*, 453–460. [CrossRef]
112. Health Canada, Eating Well with Canada's Food Guide. 2007. Available online: http://www.hc-sc.gc.ca/fn-an/food-guide-aliment/index-eng.php (accessed on 9 December 2021).
113. Chatterton, M.L.; Mihalopoulos, C.; O'Neil, A.; Itsiopoulos, C.; Opie, R.; Castle, D.; Dash, S.; Brazionis, L.; Berk, M.; Jacka, F. Economic evaluation of a dietary intervention for adults with major depression (the "SMILES" trial). *BMC Public Health* **2018**, *18*, 599. [CrossRef] [PubMed]

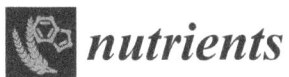

Review

The Role of Iron and Zinc in the Treatment of ADHD among Children and Adolescents: A Systematic Review of Randomized Clinical Trials

Roser Granero [1,2,3,*], Alfred Pardo-Garrido [1], Ivonne Lorena Carpio-Toro [4,5], Andrés Alexis Ramírez-Coronel [4,6], Pedro Carlos Martínez-Suárez [4,6] and Geovanny Genaro Reivan-Ortiz [3,4]

[1] Department of Psychobiology and Methodology, Autonomous University of Barcelona, 08193 Barcelona, Spain; Alfredo.Pardo@uab.cat
[2] Ciber Fisiopatología Obesidad y Nutrición (CIBERobn), Instituto Salud Carlos III, 28029 Madrid, Spain
[3] Basic Psychology, Behavioral Analysis and Programmatic Development PAD-Group, Catholic University of Cuenca, Cuenca 010107, Ecuador; greivano@ucacue.edu.ec
[4] Laboratory of Basic Psychology, Behavioral Analysis and Programmatic Development PAD-Lab, Catholic University of Cuenca, Cuenca 010107, Ecuador; icarpiot@ucacue.edu.ec (I.L.C.-T.); andres.ramirez@ucacue.edu.ec (A.A.R.-C.); pmartinezs@ucacue.edu.ec (P.C.M.-S.)
[5] Laboratory of Psychometry, Comparative Psychology and Ethology, Catholic University of Cuenca, Cuenca 010107, Ecuador
[6] Health and Behavior Research Group (HBR), Catholic University of Cuenca, Cuenca 010107, Ecuador
* Correspondence: Roser.Granero@uab.cat

Abstract: Attention-deficit/hyperactivity disorder (ADHD) is a neurodevelopmental disorder common from childhood to adulthood, affecting 5% to 12% among the general population in developed countries. Potential etiological factors have been identified, including genetic causes, environmental elements and epigenetic components. Nutrition is currently considered an influencing factor, and several studies have explored the contribution of restriction and dietary supplements in ADHD treatments. Iron is an essential cofactor required for a number of functions, such as transport of oxygen, immune function, cellular respiration, neurotransmitter metabolism (dopamine production), and DNA synthesis. Zinc is also an essential trace element, required for cellular functions related to the metabolism of neurotransmitters, melatonin, and prostaglandins. Epidemiological studies have found that iron and zinc deficiencies are common nutritional deficits worldwide, with important roles on neurologic functions (poor memory, inattentiveness, and impulsiveness), finicky appetite, and mood changes (sadness and irritability). Altered levels of iron and zinc have been related with the aggravation and progression of ADHD. Objective: This is a systematic review focused on the contribution of iron and zinc in the progression of ADHD among children and adolescents, and how therapies including these elements are tolerated along with its effectiveness (according to PRISMA guidelines). Method: The scientific literature was screened for randomized controlled trials published between January 2000 to July 2021. The databases consulted were Medline, PsycINFO, Web of Science, and Google Scholar. Two independent reviewers screened studies, extracted data, and assessed quality and risk of bias (CONSORT, NICE, and Cochrane checklists used). Conclusion: Nine studies met the eligibility criteria and were selected. Evidence was obtained regarding the contribution of iron-zinc supplementation in the treatment of ADHD among young individuals. The discussion was focused on how the deficits of these elements contribute to affectation on multiple ADHD correlates, and potential mechanisms explaining the mediational pathways. Evidence also suggested that treating ADHD with diet interventions might be particularly useful for specific subgroups of children and adolescents, but further investigations of the effects of these diet interventions are needed.

Keywords: ADHD; zinc; iron; treatment; children

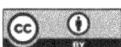

1. Introduction

Attention-deficit hyperactivity disorder (ADHD) is a neurodevelopmental disorder, usually beginning in early childhood and with a chronic progression to adulthood with several negative consequences, such as low self-esteem, difficulties in interpersonal relationships, and problems in school learning [1]. Subtypes according to the Diagnostic and Statistical Manual of Mental Disorders (5th edition) are inattention (being unable to keep focus), hyperactivity (excess movement that is not fitting to the setting) and impulsivity (hasty acts that occur without thought) [2]. Epidemiological studies indicate that ADHD is one of the most common mental disorders affecting children [3,4], with prevalence in the childhood–adolescent community ranging between 2% and 8% globally [5,6]. High prevalence rates persist in adult ADHD patients, into the range of 2.6% to 6.8% [7,8].

Etiological research outlines that ADHD constitutes a complex condition with multiple interactive factors [9]. Specific causes of the disorder are yet to be determined, but various contributing risk factors have been identified, including genetics [10–13], epigenetics [14,15], problems during pregnancy (such as stress, substance use, and other mental and physical diseases) [16–18], premature birth [19,20], obstetric and neonatal complications [21–24], and infections [25,26]. Neuropsychological mechanisms have also been identified in the onset and course of ADHD, such as brain injuries [27], neuroanatomical substrates related with genuine motor dysfunction [28] and deficient decision-making [29]. Diet-related factors (such as vitamin and/or mineral deficiencies) have also been evidenced to contribute to the levels of ADHD and the progression of the disease [30–32].

Diverse treatment plans have demonstrated to improve the symptoms of ADHD, usually combining medication (stimulants and non-stimulants have proved efficacy) with behavioral therapy [33,34]. Empirical-based pharmacological plans that have been used for decades include methylphenidate, amphetamine, atomoxetine, and guanfacine [35,36]. However, some children using these medications only experience partial relief of symptoms, which persist even with a change in medication or adjustment in dose [37]. Additionally, a number of patients with medication report significant adverse effects, such as loss of appetite, irritability, and sleep disorders [38,39]. Other typical ADHD correlates, such as restless leg syndrome, also persist despite medication [40,41].

On the other hand, despite growing pharmacological discoveries, mental disorders (such as ADHD) have shown a gradual rise during the last few decades, and rates are expected to continue increasing in the coming years [42–44]. Interestingly, it has been observed that worsening mental health within developed countries could be related to diet habits (more precisely, to the transition to more calorically dense ones) and to lower levels of physical activity [45]. Centered in the area of ADHD, various studies have shown harmful effects of the diet in the onset and progression of ADHD, including the use of preservatives and food additives [46,47]. Within this research area, it has also been observed that changes in the diet style could improve treatment efficiency for ADHD, particularly the utilization of some minerals and vitamins [48].

Dietary models have proved to be relevant to both metabolic performance and individuals' behavior. Restriction and elimination diets have been tested in ADHD treatments [49], and supplements and nutritional products have also been used as complementary intervention plans [50,51]. Studies assessing the specific role of iron and zinc on the course of ADHD have observed the deficiency of both minerals in most cases of hyperactivity [52]. Zinc is an essential mineral involved in numerous cellular metabolic processes, required for the catalytic activity of a large number of enzymes, implied in the accurate functioning of the immune system and with a role in the protein synthesis, DNA synthesis, and cell division [53]. Zinc also contributes to normal growth and development from pregnancy to adolescence, and harmonizes the performance of dopamine and melatonin [54]. Iron is a cofactor mineral that systematizes the production of dopamine and norepinephrine, an essential element participating in a wide variety of metabolic processes, including oxygen transport, deoxyribonucleic acid synthesis, and electron transport [55].

Some studies have analyzed the contribution of zinc and iron on ADHD occurrence, but conflicting findings have been obtained [56]. As a trend, compared to healthy control groups, lower levels of iron and zinc have been observed in children diagnosed with ADHD, but it is not clear whether changes in nutrient levels in blood tests mediate treatment outcomes in children with ADHD who consume mineral supplements [57,58], or even what sub-groups could particularly benefit from.

On the basis of the controversial results published regarding the role of dietary nutrients with zinc and iron for the treatment of ADHD [59,60], we performed this qualitative systematic review aimed to provide an updated account of the evidence published in randomized clinical trials assessing the efficacy of both supplements in the treatment of ADHD among children and adolescents.

2. Materials and Methods

2.1. Procedure

This systematic review was done in accordance with the eligible criteria reported in the *Preferred Reporting Items for Systematic Reviews and Meta-Analysis* (PRISMA) [61] (see Table S1, Supplementary Material), the *Assessment of Multiple Systematic Review* (AMSTAR) [62] and the *Cochrane Handbook for Systematic Reviews of Interventions* [63].

2.2. Inclusion and Exclusion Criteria

Medline, PsychINFO, Web of Science, and Google Scholar databases were searched. The search was further limited to the next inclusion criteria: (1) studies which examined treatments for ADHD; (2) which were based on randomized-controlled clinical trials; (3) which were published in English/Spanish language; (4) which were published in peer-reviewed Journals between January 2000 and July 2021; (5) which aimed to assess the efficacy of a nutritional intervention through iron or zinc supplementation; (6) which assessed clinical samples of ADHD patients diagnosed according to the Diagnostic and Statistical Manual of Mental Disorders (DSM) criteria, the 4th [64] or 5th [2] versions; (7) which analyzed participants with an age range between 5 to 18 years old; and (8) which used validated self-report instruments for measuring ADHD-related problems before and after treatment.

Specifically excluded from this systematic review were non-pill-based treatment modalities, such as behavioral interventions, neurofeedback, restriction, or alternative food exclusion diets or chiropractic interventions. No restrictions were considered for the longitudinal follow-up and interventions for the control group.

2.3. Research and Selection of Studies

The research was conducted on 20 July 2021. The strategy research (keywords and search sequence) for each database was:

- Medline: search = [((zinc OR iron) AND (ADHD)) AND ((treatment or therapy))]. The next filters were employed: (a) type of publication: (Clinical Trial) and (Randomized Controlled Trial); and (b) Date of publication: (From 1 January 2000–31 July 2021).
- PsycINFO: search = [((zinc OR iron) AND (ADHD)) AND ((treatment or therapy))]. The next filters were defined: (a) Type of publication: [Peer Reviewed Journal]; and (b) Date of publication: [1 January 2000–31 July 2021];
- Web of Science: search = [(((zinc OR iron OR ferritin) AND (ADHD)) AND ((treatment or therapy))))]. The next filters were defined: (a) Document Types: [Clinical Trial], and (b) Publication years: [1 January 2000–31 July 2021];
- Google Scholar: search = [(zinc OR iron) AND (supplement) AND (ADHD) AND (treatment or therapy) AND (randomized or "clinical trial") AND (children or adolescent) AND ("Peer Reviewed Journal")].

Two authors of this systematic review independently analyzed the title and abstract of each record, according to the inclusion/exclusion criteria. Only studies meeting the eligibility criteria were then extracted. Data validation was discussed by the same authors, and disagreements were resolved by discussion and if needed by consulting a third team member until a consensus was reached.

The authors also extracted data of the identified screening records to be described and evaluated in the results section. The information considered for applying the eligibility criteria was: the date and location of publication, type of publication, sample size, participants' sex and age range, study design, type and duration of the treatment, and measures and outcomes (changes in the ADHD status, metabolic levels, and other psychological areas).

2.4. Study Quality Assessment

The *Consolidated Standards of Reporting Trials* guidelines were employed (CONSORT-2010) [65]) for assessing the study quality. This checklist is used worldwide to improve reported randomized controlled clinical trials through a list of 25 items for assessing the title (inclusion of the design type), elaboration of the abstract (structured and completed), background and explanation of the rationale, definition of the objectives and hypothesis, description of the trial design (including important changes to methods after trial commencement and reasons), eligibility criteria for participants, the setting and location where the data were collected, intervention description (sufficient details to allow replication), completely defined outcome measures, sample size calculation (or power analysis), the method used to generate the random allocation sequence (including type of randomization), use of blinding methods, statistical procedures used for the analyses, results description (including comparison at baseline), discussion of the results (including limitations and generalizability), and other information (registration, protocol, and funding).

In addition, two checklists were used. First, the guidance elaborated by the National Institute for Health and Care Excellence: The NICE Methodology Checklist for Randomized Controlled Trials [66], which includes items structured in four sections: (a) assessment of the selection bias (appropriate method of randomization used, adequate concealment of allocation and comparability at baseline); (b) assessment of the performance bias (the comparison groups received the same care apart from the interventions, and using double-blind method); (c) assessment of the attrition bias (the groups followed for an equal length of time, and comparable treatment completion); and (d) assessment of detection bias (adequate length of follow-up, use of precise definition for the outcomes, valid and reliable methods for measuring the outcomes and triple-blind method used). Second, the Critical Appraisal Skills Programme (CASP) Randomized Controlled Trial Standard Checklist [67], which includes a set of items organized in four sections: (a) validity of the study design (clearly focused research question, randomized assignment of the participants to groups and complete follow-up); (b) using adequate methodology procedures (blinded methods, similarity between the groups at the start of the controlled trial, and groups receiving the same level of care); (c) results reported comprehensively, including the estimate of the effect sizes and carrying out a cost-effectiveness analysis cost; and 4) applicability of the results (generalization features and value provided by the intervention).

The risk of bias was also assessed using the Cochrane Risk of Bias 2 checklist [68], based on seven domains: (a) the randomization process, (b) deviations from intended intervention/s, (c) missing outcome data, (d) outcome measurement/s, (e) selection of the reported results, (f) incomplete reporting, and (g) power calculation (or sample size justification).

The assessment of the methodological quality was rated by authors of this systematic review, and discrepancies were discussed and solved.

3. Results

3.1. Descriptive for the Selected Studies

The number of studies identified through database-searching was $n = 123$. After removing duplicate articles, $n = 97$ studies were screened and $n = 9$ were finally selected on the basis of the title-abstract and the eligibility criteria (Figure 1 contains the search flow-chart).

The randomized clinical trials included in the synthesis reported data for ADHD samples of children and adolescents aged 5 to 15 years old. Zinc sulfate was administered in $n = 5$ studies, iron in $n = 2$ studies, and multi-supplements containing both compounds in a $n = 2$ study. Clinical improvement was verified using standardized measurement tools for versions for parents, teachers, and/or children. Laboratory blood screening tests were also applied (at least) at baseline and at the end of the treatment.

Table 1 includes the description of the $n = 9$ randomized controlled trials of supplements with zinc and iron for the treatment of ADHD, such as: identification of the study, sample size (N), supplement administered to the experimental group, age range and mean, gender distribution, duration of the study, and the standardized measures employed for measuring the ADHD symptoms, and other related problems.

3.2. Assessment of the Methodological Quality, Adherence and Competence

Tables 2–4 contains the results of the assessment with the CONSORT, NICE, and CASP checklists for the $n = 9$ selected studies included in the systematic review. Many studies met most of the criteria. The most incomplete items were the calculation of the sample size (or the power estimation based on the sample size of the groups), carrying out a triple-blinded study [the selected studies were double-blinded (patients and researchers were unaware of whether the treatment was administered), but it was not reported whether the team analyzing the data was also unaware of which groups' data they were evaluating], obtaining the precision of the estimates (through confidence intervals or other alternative standardized effect size measures) and carrying out a cost-effectiveness analysis cost).

3.3. Assessment of the Risk of Bias of the Included Studies

Table 5 shows the risk of bias summary of the included studies. The signaling question "bias arising from the randomization process" was identified with a moderate risk of bias for all the studies because the allocation sequence was not clearly concealed in the selected studies. The signaling item "statistical power calculation" was judged as low because studies did not justify the sample size before the results section.

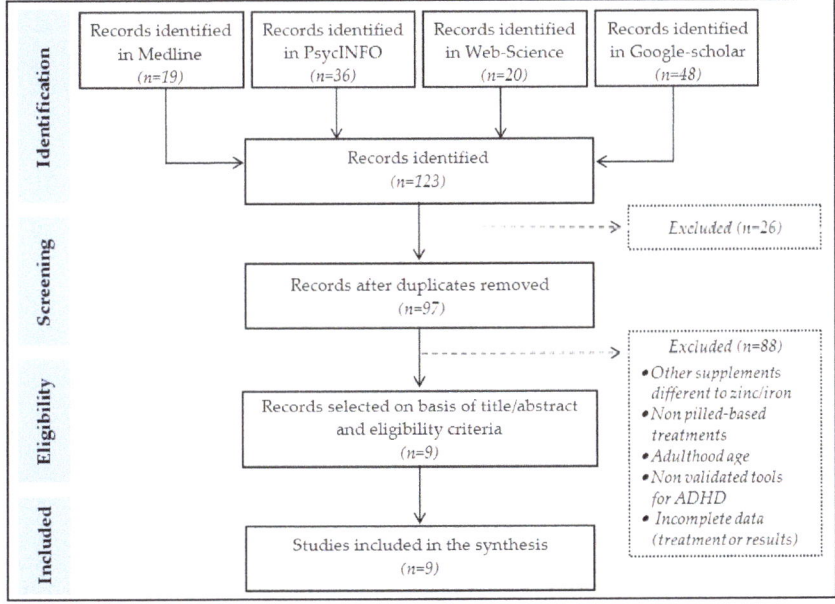

Figure 1. Search flow-chart.

Table 1. Randomized controlled trials of supplements with iron and zinc for ADHD.

Study	Refer.	N	Supp.	Dose	Age (Years)	Sex	Duration	Measures for ADHD	Results
1. Noorazar et al. (2020)	[69]	60	Zinc	10 mg zinc/day	Range = 7–12 Mean = 9.67	20% Women 80% Men	6 weeks	• Conners Parent's Questionnaire.	Zinc related with improvement, but only in the inattention factor
2. Zamora et al. (2011)	[70]	40	Zinc	10 mg zinc/day	Range = 7–14 Mean = 9.8	22.5% Women 77.5% Men	6 weeks	• Conners Rating Scales-Revised.	Improvement in the Conner's score, but only for the teacher version
3. Arnold et al. (2011)	[71]	52	Zinc	15 mg zinc/day	Range = 6–14 Mean = 9.8	17.3% Women 82.7% Men	13 weeks	• Childen's Interview for Psychiatric Syndromes (parent version). • Parent and teacher behavioral ratings. • Clinical Global Impressions (CGI). • Conners' Parent Rating Scale • Neuropsychological cognitive-motor test battery.	Equivocal results for most measures. Only neuropsychological measures mostly favored zinc
4. Akhondzadeh et al. (2004)	[72]	44	Zinc	15 mg zinc/day	Range = 5–11 Mean = 7.9	40.9% Women 59.1% Men	6 weeks	• ADH Rating Scale (ADHD-RS).	Parent and Teacher rating scale scores improved with zinc
5. Bilici et al. (2004)	[73]	400	Zinc	40 mg zinc/day	Range = 6–14 Mean = 9.6	18% Women 82% Men	12 weeks	• Attention Deficit Hyperactivity Disorder Scale (ADHDS) • Conners Teacher Questionnaire • DuPaul Parent Ratings of ADHD	Zinc related with improvements in hyperactive, impulsive and socialization symptoms. No impact of zinc was observed for the attention deficit levels. A moderator effect with age and BMI was observed
6. Konofal et al. (2008)	[74]	22	Iron	80 mg/day (ferrous sulfate, Tardyferon)	Range = 5–8 Mean = 5.9	21.7% Women 78.3% Men	12 weeks	• Conners' Parent Rating Scale • Conners' Teacher Rating Scale • Attention Deficit Hyperactivity Disorder Rating Scale (ADHD RS). • Clinical Global Impression-Severity (CGI-S).	Iron related to improvement on the ADHD RS scale and the CGI-S score. Iron did not achieved improvements on the Conner's tests

Table 1. Cont.

Study	Refer.	N	Supp.	Dose	Age (Years)	Sex	Duration	Measures for ADHD	Results
7. Panahandeh et al. (2017)	[75]	42	Iron	5 mg/kg/day (ferrous sulfate)	Range = 5–15 Mean = 8.9	9.5% Women 90.5% Men	8 weeks	• Child Symptom Inventory-4 (CSI-4).	Iron related with higher decreases on the CSI-4 total and factor scores
8. Rucklidge et al. (2018)	[76]	93	Zinc-Iron	Zinc (3.2 mg/capsule) Iron (0.9 mg/capsule). Dose: starting 3 and increasing to 12 capsules/day	Range = 5–15 Mean = 9.7	23.7% Women 76.3% Men	10 weeks	• Conners' Parent Rating Scale (CPRS-R) • Strengths and Difficulties Questionnaire (SDQ, Parents version) • Strengths and Difficulties Questionnaire (SDQ, Teachers version)	Supplements related with improvements in inattentive levels. No contribution were observed on hyperactive-impulsive symptoms.
9. Rucklidge et al. (2021)	[58]	38	Zinc-Iron	Zinc (3.2 mg/capsule) Iron (0.9 mg/capsule). Dose: starting 3 and increasing to 12 capsules/day	Range = 7–13 Mean = 10.1	21% Women 79% Men	10 weeks	• ADH Rating Scale IV (ADHD-RS-IV). • Children's Depression Rating Scale (CDRS) • Children's Globabl Assessment Scale (CGAS)	Differences in the ferritin levels achieved an interaction role for improving the ADHD severity levels.

Note: N = sample size. Supplem: supplement administered in the experimental Group. Refer: cite of the study. Dose: dosage for the supplement (zinc and iron). Results: related with the supplement (zinc and iron).

Table 2. Assessment of the studies' quality based on the CONSORT checklist.

			Title: Includes Design Type	Abstract: Structured-Complete	Introduction: Background	Introduction: Objectives-Hypothesis	Methods: Design Described	Methods: Participants	Methods: Interventions	Methods: Outcomes	Methods: Sample-Size calculation—Power	Methods: Randomization	Methods: Implementation	Methods: Statistical Procedure	Results: Participants Flow	Results: Numbers Analyzed	Results: Outcomes-Estimates	Discussion: Limitations	Discussion: Generalization	Discussion: Interpretation	Other Registration-Protocol-Funding
1.	Noorazar et al. (2020)	[69]	(+)	(+)	(+)	(P)	(+)	(+)	(+)	(+)		(+)	(+)	(+)	(+)	(+)	(P)	(+)	(P)	(+)	(+)
2.	Zamora et al. (2011)	[70]	(?)	(+)	(+)	(P)	(+)	(+)	(+)	(+)		(+)	(+)	(+)	(+)	(+)	(P)	(?)	(P)	(+)	(+)
3.	Arnold et al. (2011)	[71]	(+)	(+)	(+)	(+)	(+)	(+)	(+)	(+)		(+)	(+)	(+)	(+)	(+)	(+)	(+)	(P)	(+)	(+)
4.	Akhondzadeh et al. (2004)	[72]	(+)	(+)	(+)	(P)	(+)	(+)	(+)	(+)		(+)	(+)	(+)	(+)	(+)	(+)	(+)	(P)	(+)	(+)
5.	Bilici et al. (2004)	[73]	(+)	(+)	(+)	(+)	(+)	(+)	(+)	(+)		(+)	(+)	(+)	(+)	(P)	(P)	(?)	(P)	(+)	(+)
6.	Konofal et al. (2008)	[74]	(?)	(+)	(+)	(+)	(+)	(+)	(+)	(+)		(+)	(+)	(+)	(+)	(+)	(+)	(+)	(P)	(+)	(+)
7.	Panahandeh et al. (2017)	[75]	(?)	(+)	(+)	(P)	(+)	(+)	(+)	(+)		(+)	(+)	(+)	(+)	(+)	(+)	(+)	(P)	(+)	(+)
8.	Rucklidge et al. (2018)	[76]	(+)	(+)	(+)	(P)	(+)	(+)	(+)	(+)		(+)	(+)	(+)	(+)	(+)	(+)	(+)	(P)	(+)	(+)
9.	Rucklidge et al. (2021)	[58]	(?)	(+)	(+)	(P)	(+)	(+)	(+)	(+)		(+)	(+)	(+)	(+)	(+)	(+)	(+)	(P)	(+)	(+)

Note. (+) Green color cell: presented-reported. (P) Grey color cell: partially presented or reported with some limitations. (?) White color cell: not present or not reported.

Table 3. Assessment of the studies' quality based on the NICE checklist.

			A1. Adequate Randomization Method	A2. Adequate Concealment of Allocation	A3. Groups Comparable at Baseline	B1. Comparison Groups Received Same Care	B2. Participants Receiving Care Blind to Treatment	B3. Individuals Administering Care Blind to Allocation	C1. All Groups Followed Up for Equal Length of Time	C2a. How Many Participants Did Not Complete Treatment	C2b. Groups Comparable for Treatment Completion	C3. Participants in Each Were No Outcome Data Available	C3b. Groups Comparable Respect Availability of Outcome Data	D1. Adequate Length of Follow-Up	D2. Precise Definition of Outcome	D3. Reliable Method Used to Determine the Outcome	D4. Investigators Kept Blind to Participants Exposure	D5. Investigators Were Kept Blind to Confounding-Predictors
1.	Noorazar et al. (2020)	[69]	(+)	(+)	(+)	(+)	(+)	(+)	(+)	(+)	(+)	(+)	(+)	(+)	(+)	(+)	(?)	(?)
2.	Zamora et al. (2011)	[70]	(+)	(+)	(+)	(+)	(+)	(+)	(+)	(+)	(+)	(+)	(+)	(+)	(+)	(+)	(?)	(?)
3.	Arnold et al. (2011)	[71]	(+)	(+)	(+)	(+)	(+)	(+)	(+)	(+)	(+)	(+)	(+)	(+)	(+)	(+)	(?)	(?)
4.	Akhondzadeh et al. (2004)	[72]	(+)	(+)	(+)	(+)	(+)	(+)	(+)	(+)	(+)	(+)	(+)	(+)	(+)	(+)	(?)	(?)
5.	Bilici et al. (2004)	[73]	(+)	(+)	(?)	(+)	(+)	(+)	(+)	(+)	(+)	(+)	(+)	(+)	(+)	(+)	(?)	(?)
6.	Konofal et al. (2008)	[74]	(+)	(+)	(+)	(+)	(+)	(+)	(+)	(+)	(+)	(+)	(+)	(+)	(+)	(+)	(?)	(?)
7.	Panahandeh et al. (2017)	[75]	(+)	(+)	(+)	(+)	(+)	(+)	(+)	(+)	(+)	(+)	(+)	(+)	(+)	(+)	(?)	(?)
8.	Rucklidge et al. (2018)	[76]	(+)	(+)	(+)	(+)	(+)	(+)	(+)	(+)	(+)	(+)	(+)	(+)	(+)	(+)	(?)	(?)
9.	Rucklidge et al. (2021)	[58]	(+)	(+)	(+)	(+)	(+)	(+)	(+)	(+)	(+)	(+)	(+)	(+)	(+)	(+)	(?)	(?)

Note. (+) Green color cell: presented-reported. (?) White color cell: not present or not reported. Items A1 to A3: selection bias (systematic differences between the comparison groups). Items B1 to B3: performance bias (systematic differences between groups in the care provided, apart from the intervention under investigation). Items C1 to C3b: Attrition bias (systematic differences between the comparison groups with respect to loss of participants). Items D1 to D5: Detection bias (bias in how outcomes are ascertained, diagnosed or verified).

Table 4. Assessment of the studies' quality based on the CASP checklist.

			A1. Clearly Focused Question	A2. Use of Randomization Method	A3. Participants Accounted for	B4. Use of "Blinded" Methods	B5. Groups Similar at the Start of Randomization	B6. Each Study Group Received the Same Care	C7. Effects of Intervention Adequately Reported	C8. Precision Estimates Reported (CI or Other Effect Sizes)	C9. Cost-Effectiveness Analysis Was Done	D10. Applicability of the Results	D11. Intervention Provides Value
1.	Noorazar et al. (2020)	[69]	(+)	(+)	(+)	(+)	(+)	(+)	(+)	(?)	(?)	(+)	(+)
2.	Zamora et al. (2011)	[70]	(+)	(+)	(+)	(+)	(+)	(+)	(+)	(?)	(?)	(+)	(+)
3.	Arnold et al. (2011)	[71]	(+)	(+)	(+)	(+)	(+)	(+)	(+)	(+)	(?)	(+)	(+)
4.	Akhondzadeh et al. (2004)	[72]	(+)	(+)	(+)	(+)	(+)	(+)	(+)	(?)	(?)	(+)	(+)
5.	Bilici et al. (2004)	[73]	(+)	(+)	(+)	(+)	(+)	(?)	(+)	(?)	(?)	(+)	(+)
6.	Konofal et al. (2008)	[74]	(+)	(+)	(+)	(+)	(+)	(+)	(+)	(+)	(?)	(+)	(+)
7.	Panahandeh et al. (2017)	[75]	(+)	(+)	(+)	(+)	(+)	(+)	(+)	(?)	(?)	(+)	(+)
8.	Rucklidge et al. (2018)	[76]	(+)	(+)	(+)	(+)	(+)	(+)	(+)	(+)	(?)	(+)	(+)
9.	Rucklidge et al. (2021)	[58]	(+)	(+)	(+)	(+)	(+)	(+)	(+)	(+)	(?)	(+)	(+)

Note. (+) Green color cell: present-reported; (?) White color cell: not present or not reported. Items A1 to A3: the study design is valid for a randomized controlled trial. Items B4 to B6: the study methodology is sound. Items C7 to C9: the results are adequately reported. Items D10 to D11: the interpretation of the results is helpful.

Table 5. Assessment of the risk of bias based on the Cochrane Risk of Bias 2 checklist.

			Randomization	Deviations from the Intended Intervention/s	Missing Outcome Data	Outcome Measurements	Selective Reporting	Incomplete Reporting	Study Power Calculation/Sample Size Justification
1.	Noorazar et al. (2020)	[69]	(?)	(+)	(+)	(+)	(+)	(+)	(−)
2.	Zamora et al. (2011)	[70]	(?)	(+)	(+)	(+)	(+)	(+)	(−)
3.	Arnold et al. (2011)	[71]	(?)	(+)	(+)	(+)	(+)	(+)	(−)
4.	Akhondzadeh et al. (2004)	[72]	(?)	(+)	(+)	(+)	(+)	(+)	(−)
5.	Bilici et al. (2004)	[73]	(?)	(+)	(+)	(+)	(+)	(+)	(−)
6.	Konofal et al. (2008)	[74]	(?)	(+)	(+)	(+)	(+)	(+)	(−)
7.	Panahandeh et al. (2017)	[75]	(?)	(+)	(+)	(+)	(+)	(+)	(−)
8.	Rucklidge et al. (2018)	[76]	(?)	(+)	(+)	(+)	(+)	(+)	(−)
9.	Rucklidge et al. (2021)	[58]	(?)	(+)	(+)	(+)	(+)	(+)	(−)

Note. (+) Green color cell: low risk of bias. (?) Grey color cell: moderate risk of bias (unclear reporting or partially reported). (−) Brown color cell: high risk of bias (non-reported). Randomization: low bias judged if both a method of randomization and concealing allocation was clearly described, along with no clear obvious baseline differences between groups. Deviation: low bias judged if study participants did not change between groups. Missing outcome: low bias judged if less than 20% of participants were lost between the beginning and the end of the treatment. Outcome measurement: low bias judged if validated tools were used for the main results (e.g., standardized questionnaires). Selective reporting: low bias judged if outcomes were pre-specified. Incomplete reporting: low bias judged if measurement methods, procedure, analysis and outcomes were specified in advance to the results section. Power calculation/sample size justification: low bias judged if this was performed in advance and attained in the study.

3.4. Efficacy of Zinc for ADHD Treatment

The study of Noorazar and colleagues used the next intervention [69]: (a) a dose of 0.5–1 mg/kg/day methylphenidate plus placebo in the control group; and (b) a dose of 0.5–1 mg/kg/day methylphenidate plus 10 mg zinc (10 cc zinc sulfate syrup). No differences between the groups were observed regarding the dose of methylphenidate. After 6 weeks of treatment, the authors found that the use of zinc was useful to decrease the inattention scores ($p = 0.02$), but no differences between the groups were found in the other measures for the hyperactivity and impulsivity scales. The lack of differences in the total ADHD score in this study suggested that augmentation with zinc could only partially improve ADHD severity levels. The authors of the study also noticed that the difference between the two groups regarding the gender ratio compromised the generalization capacity, and that the use of the Connors Parent's Questionnaire as the only measure for ADHD was a significant limitation [although it is a standardized tool, the inclusion of additional instruments and informants (such as teachers) could have provided different perspectives of the children's behaviors and impairments].

The study of Zamora and colleagues also valued the effect of zinc supplementation (10 mg/day) as an adjuvant therapy (complementary to methylphenidate, with a dose of 0.3 mg/kg/day) for ADHD in $n = 40$ pediatric children, and obtained an improvement in ADHD signs associated to the experimental group in the questionnaires answered by teachers (no differences emerged from the parents' reports) [70]. These authors also obtained decreased zinc levels during the intervention in both groups (control and experimental conditions), suggesting that the methylphenidate could contribute to a decrease in zinc concentration that can be counteracted with zinc supplementation.

In the research by Arnold et al. with $n = 52$ ADHD children treated with d-amphetamine (weight-standardized) and zinc complementation (15 mg/day or 30 mg/day) or d-amphetamine and a placebo, a similar improvement in ADHD was observed in all the conditions (more precisely, teachers' ratings showed medium effect sizes favoring zinc, but parents' reports showed an opposite trend favoring the placebo) [71]. Interestingly, this trial also observed that the group treated with 30 mg/day zinc obtained 37% lower plasma levels of conventional drugs. The authors of this trial concluded that rises in zinc levels in blood tests suggested that children with ADHD may have a zinc-wasting metabolism (defined as low levels of zinc related with potential deficits in absorption or losses in urine), and therefore the zinc administered in the morning acted only as an immediate-release stimulant (this was probably the reason of the teachers' reports favoring this dietary supplement) but was next immediately excreted by mid-afternoon (parents could not observe improvements on the children's behaviors). As a global conclusion, Arnold and colleagues indicated that their study did not support zinc supplementation as a complementary tool for ADHD treatments, but also suggested that before discarding zinc as a potential treatment, it would be desirable that future research explores the situation further with different zinc doses/preparations, samples with children characterized for low zinc levels, and measures focused on neuropsychological tests as primary outcomes.

The study carried out by Akhondzadeh et al. aimed to compare two groups of patients with ADHD (with or without zinc augmentation, with a dose of approximately 15 mg/day) and both conditions treated with methylphenidate (1 mg/kg/day), and the experimental group obtained more improvement according to parents' and teachers' ratings at 6 weeks of the intervention [72]. Trend analyses also showed that differences between the groups increased during the treatment: while the placebo and the zinc supplementation groups only showed small differences at week 2, moderate to high differences were found at 4 weeks and 6 weeks (this pattern was observed for the questionnaires answered by teachers and parents).

The study by Bilici and colleagues among a large sample of $n = 400$ children with ADHD observed that the group receiving the zinc supplement (approximate dose of 40 mg/day) compared with the control group (receiving placebo) obtained greater improvements in multiple measures (hyperactivity, impulsivity, and socialization symptoms) but results were similar for attention deficiency [73]. The greatest differences between the groups were observed at 12 weeks of the intervention, and were few during 1 to 4 weeks. Regarding the potential mechanisms explaining these results, the authors conclude that the zinc supplement could affect the conversion of dietary pyridoxine to its active form (pyrodoxal phosphate), implied in the process of conversion of tryptophan to serotonin. In this sense, zinc should contribute to the increase in serotonergic functions, contributing to a decrease in the characteristic of impulsivity as a symptom of ADHD. Alternatively, the authors also suggested the existence of a synergism of zinc in regulating dopamine and norepinephrine, which has been implied in ADHD treatments. The study by Bilici et al. also showed that pre/post differences in the ADHD measures were predicted by age and BMI (a positive association was found in the B-slopes in regression analyses as higher age, and the BMI as higher change). Low pre-treatment zinc and free fatty acid values were also associated with a smaller decrease in ADHD symptom levels before and after the treatments. This evidence was also useful to determine which children could benefit more from including zinc supplementations in the ADHD treatments.

3.5. Efficacy of Iron for ADHD Treatment

The study by Konofal and colleagues aimed to examine the contribution of iron supplementation (ferrous sulfate, 80 mg/day) in a sample of n = 23 children who met the criteria for ADHD, which showed that the experimental group reported more improvement than the control group in different treatment outcomes [74]: ADHD symptom levels reported by patients, parents, and teachers (particularly marked for the inattention factor), and also the presence of restless leg syndrome. The authors did not find a correlation between the baseline levels of serum ferritin levels with endpoint ADHD measures, suggesting that children with the lowest pre-treatment ferritin values did not benefit more from iron supplementation therapy than other children. In their conclusions, these authors suggested that the effectiveness of ferrous sulfate could be associated with the ADHD pathophysiology, that the benefits of restless leg syndrome could be the consequence of the improvement in the ADHD motor activity in the evening, and that iron could enhance the action of pharmacological treatment with methylphenidate and amphetamine.

The study of Panahandeh et al. in a sample of n = 42 children with ADHD also obtained benefits for the use of ferrous sulfate (5 mg/kg/day) plus methylphenidate (1 mg/kg/day), in the inattentiveness, hyperactivity, and impulsive symptom levels reported by parents at 2 months of treatment [75]. In the conclusions section, these authors supported the hypothesis that the contribution of iron supplementation on the ADHD improvements could be explained by the capacity of this element in the dopamine transporter density and activity, which is consistent with other studies that observed decreased thalamic iron levels in children with ADHD compared to controls [77,78].

3.6. Efficacy of Including Simultaneously Iron and Zinc for ADHD Treatment

Some randomized clinical studies have also valued the contribution of multimineral-vitamin supplements which include zinc and iron for ADHD treatment in children. The rationale for selecting trails with multi-supplements therapy plans for ADHD was the low number of trails using simultaneously zinc and iron, and those identified used preparations with vitamins, dietary minerals and other nutritional elements. Therefore, considering these studies facilitates generalizability of the results related with the use of zinc–iron supplements.

The study of Rucklidge and colleagues [76] in a sample of n = 93 patients used Daily Essential Nutrients (DEN, with Recommended Dietary Allowances, RDA), which contains a comprehensive range of micronutrients (13 vitamins, 17 minerals, and 4 amino acids). The participants were instructed to titrate the dose up to over a week, starting with 3 capsules per day and increasing it to up to 12 capsules per day (see Table 1 for the zinc–iron content). This study obtained an intent-to-treat analysis of between-group differences with greater improvements for ADHD related with the micronutrient treatment, but specifically in the clinicians' reports assessing inattention. However, although no significant differences were found for the hyperactivity and impulsive measures between the experimental and the placebo groups, the micronutrients supplement obtained improvements in emotional regulation, aggression, and general functioning. The authors of this study concluded that the mechanisms of action of micronutrient treatments likely involves different pathways rather than pharmacological treatments, and that supplements like those used in the study may have an impact on the methylation/methionine cycle, required for the synthesis of DNA/RNA (as it was suggested by other studies [79]), and on the citric acid cycle and electron transport chain acting as co-enzymes in mitochondrial aerobic respiration and energy production. These potential effects on the physical state could also contribute to improvements in mood state and cognition functions (also suggested in the literature [80,81]).

Finally, the study of Rucklidge et al. was published later and carried out on a sample of n = 38 children that also used DEN, with an initial dose of 3 capsules per day which further increased to 12 capsules per day (see Table 1 for the zinc–iron content). This study showed that a broad-spectrum micronutrient formula (EMPowerplus) served as a mediator in the treatment response considering multiple ADHD measures [58]. Interestingly, only pre/post changes in the copper and ferritin levels achieved a significant moderator role on the improvement registered for the severity of ADHD: as the increase in the ferritin and the decrease in the copper highly benefited the levels of ADHD (in the three dimensions of inattentiveness, hyperactivity, and impulsivity). However, the authors indicated that these results should be interpreted with caution, and outlined the need to consider individual variability: since metabolic needs are different between the patients, as well as their genetic makeup, some children may need certain nutrients to restore optimal metabolic functioning, and others will not require specific nutrients and should not benefit from supplementations. In addition, nutrients act in a synergistic way, and therefore, changes in one can have cascading effects on others, and it was thus unlikely that increases in a specific nutrient could make a direct and unique contribution on the changes observed in a complex disorder, such as ADHD.

3.7. Tolerability Analyses

Regarding safety and tolerability, no serious adverse events were reported in the studies selected for this review, and the unpleasant events found were similar for the experimental and control groups. Iron and zinc therapies were generally well-tolerated: no patients referred to an exacerbation of ADHD symptoms or a significant decrease in appetite, and only a low number of children reported physical pains, nausea, vomiting, constipation, or a metallic taste in the mouth. Moreover, studies suggested that maintaining a fixed daily dose of iron–zinc was a relevant factor in increasing tolerability, and no indication regarding any great concern about the doses up to the follow-up was registered. However, it cannot be determined whether a long-term zinc–iron treatment could induce negative events, such as toxicity or hemosiderosis.

4. Discussion

This study conducted a qualitative systematic review of the empirical evidence obtained in randomized clinical trials published since 2000 on the efficacy of zinc and iron supplementation among ADHD children and adolescents. Nine studies met the eligibility criteria and were selected. Results indicated that low zinc and iron levels were related with both higher baseline levels of ADHD severity and poorer treatment outcomes. Compared with the controlled-placebo conditions, the dietary supplements with zinc and iron were associated with improvements in ADHD severity at the end of the treatments, although the effect size of the outcomes tended to be low and/or focused on specific ADHD symptoms/measures.

Cross-sectional evidence regarding the association of zinc and iron with ADHD levels (pre-treatment associations) is consistent with other non-randomized studies that explored the contribution of these micronutrients within clinical- and population-based samples. For example, a longitudinal study with a large sample with $n = 608$ children found that zinc–iron supplementation improved attention/concentration in children over a 14-month follow-up period [82]. A positive correlation was also found between zinc and symptoms of inattentiveness in a cross-sectional study of $n = 48$ children [83].

The potential explanations about the paths between the zinc–iron levels and the various ADHD manifestations are discussed in a number of studies, which showed that lower levels of these elements in childhood (but also in older adults) could be related to a dopaminergic impairment, which could be the origin of the high inattentiveness–hyperactivity levels and the other correlates of the ADHD disease (like the presence of restless leg syndrome and other multiple sleep problems) [74,84,85]. Neuroimaging, genetic, and animal studies have also shown that decreases in dopamine transporter densities are related with decreased brain iron and zinc levels [86–88]. Zinc achieves a relevant role in the metabolism of neurotransmitters, prostaglandins, and for maintaining brain structure and function. Since zinc is necessary in the metabolism of melatonin, it is strongly implied in the regulation of dopamine (zinc is therefore considered a dopamine reuptake inhibitor). Iron is a cofactor in the tyrosine hydroxylase enzyme, and a key cofactor in the making of neurotransmitters, including serotonin, norepinephrine, and dopamine. Brain iron-deficient rodents have been associated with alterations in adenosine neurotransmission, which has provided a pathogenetic link with glutamate mechanisms and the hypersensitive corticostriatal terminals involved in some ADHD correlates [89,90].

The link between iron and zinc supplementation and the observed decrease in ADHD symptoms in the controlled clinical trials selected for this systematic review also makes sense with regard to the role of zinc and iron as dopamine reuptake inhibitors, which was precisely the core target of the stimulant medications used in the combined treatment plans for the disease. Other non-randomized studies using a combination of polyunsaturated fatty acids with zinc supplementation also showed benefits for the treatment of ADHD. For example, the observational study of Huss et al. in a large sample of n = 810 monitored children aged 5–12 years old showed that consumption of omega-3 and omega-6 with complementation of zinc improved ADHD symptoms, as well as other emotional problems, and sleeping disease (attention deficit, hyperactivity, and impulsivity) after 12 weeks [91]. The rationale for these results could be found in the capacity of these dietary combinations for facilitating the transmission of signals between neurons, which also contributed to improvements in attention ability, learning difficulties, and executive functions in the development of children and adolescents [92,93].

The studies included in this review support the existence of subgroups (based on the treatment outcomes and its baseline clinical correlates) that could be particularly benefitted from treatments including dietary zinc and iron supplements, such as the results of Bilici and colleagues [73]: the association found in this study between the low baseline zinc values with lower improvements in the ADHD measures suggested that zinc may be particularly important for the treatment of this disorder, improving and compensating borderline zinc nutrition. The study of Arnold and colleagues, which reanalyzed data from a randomized clinical trial with n = 18 children by comparing d-amphetamine with Efamol, assessed the moderate role of zinc [94], categorized the participants into three groups (as zinc-adequate, zinc-borderline, and zinc-deficient), and observed a linear relationship of d-amphetamine with zinc nutrition among the d-amphetamine group, and a quadratic (U-shaped) relationship of Efamol response to zinc (the benefit among this group was only found among the zinc-borderline condition). Finally, the research based on a secondary analysis of data collected in the study of Arnold and colleagues [71] analyzed the role of the status of iron, and determined that it was associated with ADHD symptom severity at baseline and with responses to psycho-stimulant treatment [95]. This study found an inverse correlation of serum ferritin with baseline inattention, hyperactivity, and impulsivity levels (as ferritin concentration increased, ADHD severity decreased), and also a significant correlation between serum ferritin and sensitivity to the amphetamine used for ADHD treatment (participants with higher ferritin concentrations required lower weight-adjusted doses of psychotropic treatment). These results were obtained after adjusting for the participants' sex and age. The authors concluded that iron supplementation could contribute as a potential intervention to optimize responses to psycho-stimulants in children with low iron stores at baseline. Other studies have also showed that ferritin concentration is correlated with the dose of amphetamine necessary to reach an optimal clinical response [96]. However, results in this area are few, and future research should address the question of which are the optimal doses, as well as the benefits of using supplements of multiple vitamins and minerals.

5. Conclusions

Based on the results obtained in this systematic review, the specific role of dietary nutrients with zinc and iron still seems controversial for the treatment of ADHD, being most consistent with the evidence for zinc. Moreover, although the reviewed studies found a relationship between the use of dietary supplements containing these elements with the improvement of ADHD symptoms, neither the mono-causal role of a concrete specific nutritional deficiency among ADHD children nor the role of a concrete dietary nutrient in the management of this disorder were proven (as was reported quite recently [56]). Future controlled clinical trials are needed, examining the efficacy of mineral supplementation.

The results obtained in this systematic review should be considered for combining these multi-facet interventions with additional precise interventions, specifically focused on the nutritional state and clinical profile of each patient. The ultimate objective of these treatments, including medical, psychological, and diet plans, should be to decrease the levels of ADHD, but also its multiple negative correlates, in order to achieve better performance in vigilance and sustained attention tasks, executive functioning tasks (like planning and organization), set shifting and response monitoring, and complex problem-solving.

Finally, this study should be interpreted in consideration of certain limitations. First, a meta-analysis was not conducted. Systematic reviews of treatment plans often include statistical methods to summarize the results of independent research by combining the information of selected studies (through meta-analysis) with the aim to provide more precise estimates of the effects of health care. However, it must be outlined that not all topics allow a meta-analysis to be conducted, and these concrete systematic reviews use alternative methods of synthesis described as "narrative synthesis". This was the case of our study: we did not employ meta-analyses because of the clinical heterogeneity of individual studies, with different intervention characteristics (for example, the iron/zinc supplements were administered in two trials within multi-supplements also including other trace elements, with different doses and/or frequency of doses, and with different durations), diverse outcome/effects measurement, different research settings, and differences in participants' features (such as age, baseline disease severity, other comorbid conditions, or sociodemographic variables). Since current studies have proven that this heterogeneity could cause significant inaccurate summary effects and associated conclusions, and thus misleading decision-markers [97], we opted to conduct a narrative synthesis in accordance with the current guidelines. Other characteristics of the individual studies selected for this review also impact on the generalizability capacity of our review: the limited samples sizes, the convenience samples (non-probability sampling methods were used), and the frequency of men compared to women.

Supplementary Materials: The following are available online at https://www.mdpi.com/article/10.3390/nu13114059/s1, Table S1: PRISMA 2020 main checklist.

Author Contributions: Conceptualization: R.G. and G.G.R.-O.; formal statistical analysis: I.L.C.-T., A.A.R.-C. and P.C.M.-S.; writing—original draft preparation: R.G. and G.G.R.-O.; writing—review and editing, I.L.C.-T., A.A.R.-C., P.C.M.-S. and A.P.-G. All authors contributed substantially to the data analysis, interpretation of data. All authors have read and agreed to the published version of the manuscript.

Funding: This research received no external funding.

Conflicts of Interest: The authors declare no conflict of interest.

References

1. Di Lorenzo, R.; Balducci, J.; Poppi, C.; Arcolin, E.; Cutino, A.; Ferri, P.; D'Amico, R.; Filippini, T. Children and adolescents with ADHD followed up to adulthood: A systematic review of long-term outcomes. *Acta Neuropsychiatr.* **2021**, 1–42. [CrossRef]
2. American Psychiatric Association. *Diagnostic and Statistical Manual of Mental Disorders: DSM-5*, 5th ed.; American Psychiatric Association: Washington, DC, USA, 2013.
3. Chan, M.F.; Al Balushi, R.; Al Falahi, M.; Mahadevan, S.; Al Saadoon, M.; Al-Adawi, S. Child and adolescent mental health disorders in the GCC: A systematic review and meta-analysis. *Int. J. Pediatr. Adolesc. Med.* **2021**, *8*, 134–145. [CrossRef] [PubMed]
4. Polanczyk, G.V.; Salum, G.A.; Sugaya, L.S.; Caye, A.; Rohde, L.A. Annual Research Review: A meta-analysis of the worldwide prevalence of mental disorders in children and adolescents. *J. Child Psychol. Psychiatry* **2015**, *56*, 345–365. [CrossRef]
5. Sayal, K.; Prasad, V.; Daley, D.; Ford, T.; Coghill, D. ADHD in children and young people: Prevalence, care pathways, and service provision. *Lancet Psychiatry* **2018**, *5*, 175–186. [CrossRef]
6. Willis, R.; Dhakras, S.; Cortese, S. Attention-Deficit/Hyperactivity Disorder in Looked-After Children: A Systematic Review of the Literature. *Curr. Dev. Disord. Rep.* **2017**, *4*, 78–84. [CrossRef] [PubMed]
7. Dobrosavljevic, M.; Solares, C.; Cortese, S.; Andershed, H.; Larsson, H. Prevalence of attention-deficit/hyperactivity disorder in older adults: A systematic review and meta-analysis. *Neurosci. Biobehav. Rev.* **2020**, *118*, 282–289. [CrossRef]

8. Song, P.; Zha, M.; Yang, Q.; Zhang, Y.; Li, X.; Rudan, I. The prevalence of adult attention-deficit hyperactivity disorder: A global systematic review and meta-analysis. *J. Glob. Health* **2021**, *11*, 04009. [CrossRef]
9. Lynch, S.J.; Sunderland, M.; Newton, N.C.; Chapman, C. A systematic review of transdiagnostic risk and protective factors for general and specific psychopathology in young people. *Clin. Psychol. Rev.* **2021**, *87*, 102036. [CrossRef]
10. Bruxel, E.M.; Moreira-Maia, C.R.; Akutagava-Martins, G.C.; Quinn, T.P.; Klein, M.; Franke, B.; Ribasés, M.; Rovira, P.; Sánchez-Mora, C.; Kappel, D.B.; et al. Meta-analysis and systematic review of ADGRL3 (LPHN3) polymorphisms in ADHD susceptibility. *Mol. Psychiatry* **2020**, *26*, 2277–2285. [CrossRef] [PubMed]
11. Kang, P.; Luo, L.; Peng, X.; Wang, Y. Association of Val158Met polymorphism in COMT gene with attention-deficit hyperactive disorder: An updated meta-analysis. *Medicine* **2020**, *99*, e23400. [CrossRef]
12. McNeill, R.V.; Ziegler, G.C.; Radtke, F.; Nieberler, M.; Lesch, K.-P.; Kittel-Schneider, S. Mental health dished up—the use of iPSC models in neuropsychiatric research. *J. Neural Transm.* **2020**, *127*, 1547–1568. [CrossRef]
13. Ronald, A.; de Bode, N.; Polderman, T.J. Systematic Review: How the Attention-Deficit/Hyperactivity Disorder Polygenic Risk Score Adds to Our Understanding of ADHD and Associated Traits. *J. Am. Acad. Child Adolesc. Psychiatry* **2021**, *60*, 1234–1277. [CrossRef]
14. Schuch, V.; Utsumi, D.A.; Costa, T.V.M.M.; Kulikowski, L.D.; Muszkat, M. Attention Deficit Hyperactivity Disorder in the Light of the Epigenetic Paradigm. *Front. Psychiatry* **2015**, *6*, 126. [CrossRef]
15. Walton, E.; Pingault, J.-B.; Cecil, C.A.; Gaunt, T.R.; Relton, C.C.; Mill, J.; Barker, E.D. Epigenetic profiling of ADHD symptoms trajectories: A prospective, methylome-wide study. *Mol. Psychiatry* **2016**, *22*, 250–256. [CrossRef]
16. Han, V.X.; Patel, S.; Jones, H.F.; Nielsen, T.C.; Mohammad, S.S.; Hofer, M.J.; Gold, W.; Brilot, F.; Lain, S.J.; Nassar, N.; et al. Maternal acute and chronic inflammation in pregnancy is associated with common neurodevelopmental disorders: A systematic review. *Transl. Psychiatry* **2021**, *11*, 1–12. [CrossRef]
17. Li, L.; Lagerberg, T.; Chang, Z.; Cortese, S.; Rosenqvist, M.A.; Almqvist, C.; D'Onofrio, B.M.; Hegvik, T.-A.; Hartman, C.; Chen, Q.; et al. Maternal pre-pregnancy overweight/obesity and the risk of attention-deficit/hyperactivity disorder in offspring: A systematic review, meta-analysis and quasi-experimental family-based study. *Int. J. Epidemiol.* **2020**, *49*, 857–875. [CrossRef]
18. Qu, A.; Cao, T.; Li, Z.; Wang, W.; Liu, R.; Wang, X.; Nie, Y.; Sun, S.; Liu, X.; Zhang, X. The association between maternal perfluoroalkyl substances exposure and early attention deficit hyperactivity disorder in children: A systematic review and meta-analysis. *Environ. Sci. Pollut. Res.* **2021**, 1–16. [CrossRef]
19. Bogičević, L.; Verhoeven, M.; Van Baar, A.L. Distinct Profiles of Attention in Children Born Moderate-to-Late Preterm at 6 Years. *J. Pediatr. Psychol.* **2020**, *45*, 685–694. [CrossRef]
20. Walczak-Kozłowska, T.; Mańkowska, A.; Chrzan-Dętkoś, M.; Harciarek, M. Attentional system of very prematurely born preschoolers. *Dev. Psychol.* **2020**, *56*, 251–260. [CrossRef]
21. Carlsson, T.; Molander, F.; Taylor, M.J.; Jonsson, U.; Bölte, S. Early environmental risk factors for neurodevelopmental disorders—A systematic review of twin and sibling studies. *Dev. Psychopathol.* **2020**, *33*, 1448–1495. [CrossRef]
22. Nielsen, T.M.; Pedersen, M.V.; Milidou, I.; Glavind, J.; Henriksen, T.B. Long-term cognition and behavior in children born at early term gestation: A systematic review. *Acta Obstet. Et Gynecol. Scand.* **2019**, *98*, 1227–1234. [CrossRef]
23. Rivollier, F.; Krebs, M.-O.; Kebir, O. Perinatal Exposure to Environmental Endocrine Disruptors in the Emergence of Neurodevelopmental Psychiatric Diseases: A Systematic Review. *Int. J. Environ. Res. Public Health* **2019**, *16*, 1318. [CrossRef]
24. Serati, M.; Barkin, J.L.; Orsenigo, G.; Altamura, A.C.; Buoli, M. Research Review: The role of obstetric and neonatal complications in childhood attention deficit and hyperactivity disorder—A systematic review. *J. Child Psychol. Psychiatry* **2017**, *58*, 1290–1300. [CrossRef]
25. Kalantary, R.R.; Jaffarzadeh, N.; Rezapour, M.; Arani, M.H. Association between exposure to polycyclic aromatic hydrocarbons and attention deficit hyperactivity disorder in children: A systematic review and meta-analysis. *Environ. Sci. Pollut. Res.* **2020**, *27*, 11531–11540. [CrossRef] [PubMed]
26. Dreier, J.W.; Andersen, A.-M.N.; Hvolby, A.; Garne, E.; Andersen, P.K.; Berg-Beckhoff, G. Fever and infections in pregnancy and risk of attention deficit/hyperactivity disorder in the offspring. *J. Child Psychol. Psychiatry* **2015**, *57*, 540–548. [CrossRef]
27. Nikolas, M.A.; Nigg, J.T. Moderators of Neuropsychological Mechanism in Attention-Deficit Hyperactivity Disorder. *J. Abnorm. Child Psychol.* **2014**, *43*, 271–281. [CrossRef] [PubMed]
28. Hirjak, D.; Meyer-Lindenberg, A.; Fritze, S.; Sambataro, F.; Kubera, K.M.; Wolf, R.C. Motor dysfunction as research domain across bipolar, obsessive-compulsive and neurodevelopmental disorders. *Neurosci. Biobehav. Rev.* **2018**, *95*, 315–335. [CrossRef]
29. Schulze, M.; Coghill, D.; Lux, S.; Philipsen, A. Disentangling ADHD's Presentation-Related Decision-Making—A Meta-Analytic Approach on Predominant Presentations. *Front. Psychiatry* **2021**, *12*, 519840. [CrossRef] [PubMed]
30. Curtis, L.T.; Patel, K. Nutritional and Environmental Approaches to Preventing and Treating Autism and Attention Deficit Hyperactivity Disorder (ADHD): A Review. *J. Altern. Complement. Med.* **2008**, *14*, 79–85. [CrossRef]
31. Azadbakht, L.; Hariri, M. Magnesium, iron, and zinc supplementation for the treatment of attention deficit hyperactivity disorder: A systematic review on the recent literature. *Int. J. Prev. Med.* **2015**, *6*, 83. [CrossRef]
32. Rucklidge, J.J.; Frampton, C.M.; Gorman, B.; Boggis, A. Vitamin–mineral treatment of attention-deficit hyperactivity disorder in adults: Double-blind randomised placebo-controlled trial. *Br. J. Psychiatry* **2014**, *204*, 306–315. [CrossRef] [PubMed]
33. Shahidullah, J.D.; Carlson, J.S.; Haggerty, D.; Lancaster, B.M. Integrated care models for ADHD in children and adolescents: A systematic review. *Fam. Syst. Health* **2018**, *36*, 233–247. [CrossRef]

34. Sultan, M.A.; Pastrana, C.S.; Pajer, K.A. Shared Care Models in the Treatment of Pediatric Attention-Deficit/Hyperactivity Disorder (ADHD): Are They Effective? *Health Serv. Res. Manag. Epidemiol.* **2018**, *5*, 1–7. [CrossRef]
35. Boland, H.; DiSalvo, M.; Fried, R.; Woodworth, K.Y.; Wilens, T.; Faraone, S.V.; Biederman, J. A literature review and meta-analysis on the effects of ADHD medications on functional outcomes. *J. Psychiatr. Res.* **2020**, *123*, 21–30. [CrossRef] [PubMed]
36. Weyandt, L.; Oster, D.; Marraccini, M.E.; Gudmundsdottir, B.; Munro, B.; Zavras, B.M.; Kuhar, B. Pharmacological interventions for adolescents and adults with ADHD: Stimulant and nonstimulant medications and misuse of prescription stimulants. *Psychol. Res. Behav. Manag.* **2014**, *7*, 223–249. [CrossRef]
37. Tsujii, N.; Okada, T.; Usami, M.; Kuwabara, H.; Fujita, J.; Negoro, H.; Kawamura, M.; Iida, J.; Saito, T. Effect of Continuing and Discontinuing Medications on Quality of Life After Symptomatic Remission in Attention-Deficit/Hyperactivity Disorder: A Systematic Review and Meta-Analysis. *J. Clin. Psychiatry* **2020**, *81*, 19r13015. [CrossRef] [PubMed]
38. de la Cruz, L.F.; Simonoff, E.; McGough, J.J.; Halperin, J.M.; Arnold, L.E.; Stringaris, A. Treatment of Children with Attention-Deficit/Hyperactivity Disorder (ADHD) and Irritability: Results from the Multimodal Treatment Study of Children with ADHD (MTA). *J. Am. Acad. Child Adolesc. Psychiatry* **2014**, *54*, 62–70. [CrossRef]
39. Weiss, M.D.; Salpekar, J. Sleep Problems in the Child with Attention-Deficit Hyperactivity Disorder: Defining Aetiology and Appropriate Treatments. *CNS Drugs* **2010**, *24*, 811–828. [CrossRef]
40. Chamorro, M.; Lara, J.P.; Insa, I.; Espadas, M.; Alda-Diez, J.A. Evaluacion y tratamiento de los problemas de sueño en niños diagnosticados de trastorno por deficit de atencion/hiperactividad: Actualizacion de la evidencia [Evaluation and treatment of sleep problems in children diagnosed with attention deficit hyperactivity disorder: An update of the evidence]. *Rev. Neurol.* **2017**, *64*, 413–421.
41. DelRosso, L.M.; Mogavero, M.P.; Baroni, A.; Bruni, O.; Ferri, R. Restless Legs Syndrome in Children and Adolescents. *Child Adolesc. Psychiatr. Clin. North Am.* **2020**, *30*, 143–157. [CrossRef]
42. Baxter, A.J.; Patton, G.; Scott, K.M.; Degenhardt, L.; Whiteford, H.A. Global Epidemiology of Mental Disorders: What Are We Missing? *PLoS ONE* **2013**, *8*, e65514. [CrossRef]
43. Polanczyk, G.V.; Willcutt, E.G.; Salum, G.A.; Kieling, C.; Rohde, L.A. ADHD prevalence estimates across three decades: An updated systematic review and meta-regression analysis. *Int. J. Epidemiol.* **2014**, *43*, 434–442. [CrossRef]
44. Thomas, R.; Sanders, S.; Doust, J.; Beller, E.; Glasziou, P. Prevalence of Attention-Deficit/Hyperactivity Disorder: A Systematic Review and Meta-analysis. *Pediatrics* **2015**, *135*, e994–e1001. [CrossRef]
45. Logan, A.C.; Jacka, F.N. Nutritional psychiatry research: An emerging discipline and its intersection with global urbanization, environmental challenges and the evolutionary mismatch. *J. Physiol. Anthr.* **2014**, *33*, 1–16. [CrossRef]
46. Agostoni, C.; Nobile, M.; Ciappolino, V.; DelVecchio, G.; Tesei, A.; Turolo, S.; Crippa, A.; Mazzocchi, A.; Altamura, C.A.; Brambilla, P.; et al. The Role of Omega-3 Fatty Acids in Developmental Psychopathology: A Systematic Review on Early Psychosis, Autism, and ADHD. *Int. J. Mol. Sci.* **2017**, *18*, 2608. [CrossRef] [PubMed]
47. Nigg, J.T.; Lewis, K.; Edinger, T.; Falk, M. Meta-Analysis of Attention-Deficit/Hyperactivity Disorder or Attention-Deficit/Hyperactivity Disorder Symptoms, Restriction Diet, and Synthetic Food Color Additives. *J. Am. Acad. Child Adolesc. Psychiatry* **2012**, *51*, 86–97. [CrossRef]
48. Torp, N.M.U.; Thomsen, P.H. The use of diet interventions to treat symptoms of ADHD in children and adolescents—A systematic review of randomized controlled trials. *Nord. J. Psychiatry* **2020**, *74*, 558–568. [CrossRef] [PubMed]
49. Rytter, M.J.H.; Andersen, L.B.B.; Houmann, T.; Bilenberg, N.; Hvolby, A.; Mølgaard, C.; Michaelsen, K.F.; Lauritzen, L. Diet in the treatment of ADHD in children—A systematic review of the literature. *Nord. J. Psychiatry* **2014**, *69*, 1–18. [CrossRef] [PubMed]
50. Bloch, M.H.; Mulqueen, J. Nutritional Supplements for the Treatment of ADHD. *Child Adolesc. Psychiatr. Clin. N. Am.* **2014**, *23*, 883–897. [CrossRef]
51. Verlaet, A.A.J.; Maasakkers, C.M.; Hermans, N.; Savelkoul, H.F.J. Rationale for Dietary Antioxidant Treatment of ADHD. *Nutrients* **2018**, *10*, 405. [CrossRef]
52. Del-Ponte, B.; Quinte, G.C.; Cruz, S.; Grellert, M.; Santos, I.S. Dietary patterns and attention deficit/hyperactivity disorder (ADHD): A systematic review and meta-analysis. *J. Affect. Disord.* **2019**, *252*, 160–173. [CrossRef]
53. Maret, W.; Sandstead, H.H. Zinc requirements and the risks and benefits of zinc supplementation. *J. Trace Elem. Med. Biol.* **2006**, *20*, 3–18. [CrossRef]
54. Avcil, S.; Uysal, P.; Yenisey, Ç.; Abas, B.I. Elevated Melatonin Levels in Children With Attention Deficit Hyperactivity Disorder: Relationship to Oxidative and Nitrosative Stress. *J. Atten. Disord.* **2019**, *25*, 693–703. [CrossRef]
55. Abbaspour, N.; Hurrell, R.; Kelishadi, R. Review on iron and its importance for human health. *J. Res. Med Sci. Isfahan Univ. Med Sci.* **2014**, *19*, 164–174.
56. Robberecht, H.; Verlaet, A.A.J.; Breynaert, A.; De Bruyne, T.; Hermans, N. Magnesium, Iron, Zinc, Copper and Selenium Status in Attention-Deficit/Hyperactivity Disorder (ADHD). *Molecules* **2020**, *25*, 4440. [CrossRef]
57. Rucklidge, J.J.; Eggleston, M.J.; Darling, K.A.; Stevens, A.J.; Kennedy, M.A.; Frampton, C.M. Can we predict treatment response in children with ADHD to a vitamin-mineral supplement? An investigation into pre-treatment nutrient serum levels, MTHFR status, clinical correlates and demographic variables. *Prog. Neuro-Psychopharmacol. Biol. Psychiatry* **2018**, *89*, 181–192. [CrossRef]
58. Rucklidge, J.J.; Eggleston, M.J.F.; Boggis, A.; Darling, K.; Gorman, B.; Frampton, C.M. Do Changes in Blood Nutrient Levels Mediate Treatment Response in Children and Adults with ADHD Consuming a Vitamin–Mineral Supplement? *J. Atten. Disord.* **2019**, *25*, 1107–1119. [CrossRef]

59. Fanjiang, G.; Kleinman, E.R. Nutrition and performance in children. *Curr. Opin. Clin. Nutr. Metab. Care* **2007**, *10*, 342–347. [CrossRef]
60. Rucklidge, J.J.; Johnstone, J.; Kaplan, B.J. Nutrient supplementation approaches in the treatment of ADHD. *Expert Rev. Neurother.* **2009**, *9*, 461–476. [CrossRef]
61. Page, M.J.; McKenzie, J.E.; Bossuyt, P.M.; Boutron, I.; Hoffmann, T.C.; Mulrow, C.D.; Shamseer, L.; Tetzlaff, J.M.; Akl, E.A.; Brennan, S.E.; et al. The PRISMA 2020 statement: An updated guideline for reporting systematic reviews. *PLoS Med.* **2021**, *18*, e1003583. [CrossRef]
62. Shea, B.J.; Grimshaw, J.M.; Wells, G.A.; Boers, M.; Andersson, N.; Hamel, C.; Porter, A.C.; Tugwell, P.; Moher, D.; Bouter, L.M. Development of AMSTAR: A measurement tool to assess the methodological quality of systematic reviews. *BMC Med Res. Methodol.* **2007**, *7*, 1–7. [CrossRef] [PubMed]
63. Higgins, J.P.; Green, S. Cochrane Handbook for Systematic Reviews of Interventions Version 5.1.0. The Cochrane Collaboration. 2011. Available online: https://handbook.cochrane.org (accessed on 15 July 2021).
64. American Psychiatric Association. *Diagnostic and Statistical Manual of Mental Disorders: DSM-IV-R*; American Psychiatric Association: Washington, DC, USA, 2000.
65. Welch, R.W.; Antoine, J.-M.; Berta, J.-L.; Bub, A.; De Vries, J.; Guarner, F.; Hasselwander, O.; Hendriks, H.; Jäkel, M.; Koletzko, B.V.; et al. Guidelines for the design, conduct and reporting of human intervention studies to evaluate the health benefits of foods. *Br. J. Nutr.* **2011**, *106*, S3–S15. [CrossRef] [PubMed]
66. National Institute for Health and Care Excellence, NICE. Methods for the Development of NICE Public Health Guidance. 2012. Available online: https://www.nice.org.uk/process/pmg4/resources/methods-for-the-development-of-nice-public-health-guidance-third-edition-pdf-2007967445701 (accessed on 15 July 2021).
67. Critical Appraisal Skills Programme, CASP. Randomized Controlled Trials Checklist. 2020. Available online: https://casp-uk.net/casp-tools-checklists (accessed on 15 July 2021).
68. Sterne, J.A.C.; Savović, J.; Page, M.J.; Elbers, R.G.; Blencowe, N.S.; Boutron, I.; Cates, C.J.; Cheng, H.-Y.; Corbett, M.S.; Eldridge, S.M.; et al. RoB 2: A revised tool for assessing risk of bias in randomised trials. *BMJ* **2019**, *366*, l4898. [CrossRef]
69. Noorazar, S.G.; Malek, A.; Aghaei, S.M.; Yasamineh, N.; Kalejahi, P. The efficacy of zinc augmentation in children with attention deficit hyperactivity disorder under treatment with methylphenidate: A randomized controlled trial. *Asian J. Psychiatry* **2019**, *48*, 101868. [CrossRef] [PubMed]
70. Zamora, J.; Velásquez, A.; Troncoso, L.; Barra, P.; Guajardo, K.; Castillo-Duran, C. Zinc en la terapia del sindrome de déficit de atención e hiperactividad en niños. Un estudio controlado aleatorio preliminar [Zinc in the therapy of the atten-tion-deficit/hyperactivity disorder in children. A preliminary randomized controlled trial]. *Arch. Latinoam. Nutr.* **2011**, *61*, 242–246. [PubMed]
71. Arnold, L.E.; DiSilvestro, R.A.; Bozzolo, D.; Bozzolo, H.; Crowl, L.; Fernandez, S.; Ramadan, Y.; Thompson, S.; Mo, X.; Abdel-Rasoul, M.; et al. Zinc for Attention-Deficit/Hyperactivity Disorder: Placebo-Controlled Double-Blind Pilot Trial Alone and Combined with Amphetamine. *J. Child Adolesc. Psychopharmacol.* **2011**, *21*, 1–19. [CrossRef]
72. Akhondzadeh, S.; Mohammadi, M.-R.; Khademi, M. Zinc sulfate as an adjunct to methylphenidate for the treatment of attention deficit hyperactivity disorder in children: A double blind and randomized trial [ISRCTN64132371]. *BMC Psychiatry* **2004**, *4*, 1–6. [CrossRef]
73. Bilici, M.; Yıldırım, F.; Kandil, S.; Bekaroğlu, M.; Yıldırmış, S.; Değer, O.; Ülgen, M.; Yıldıran, A.; Aksu, H. Double-blind, placebo-controlled study of zinc sulfate in the treatment of attention deficit hyperactivity disorder. *Prog. Neuro-Psychopharmacol. Biol. Psychiatry* **2004**, *28*, 181–190. [CrossRef]
74. Konofal, E.; Lecendreux, M.; Deron, J.; Marchand, M.; Cortese, S.; Zaïm, M.; Mouren, M.C.; Arnulf, I. Effects of iron supplementation on attention deficit hyperactivity disorder in children. *Pediatr. Neurol.* **2008**, *38*, 20–26. [CrossRef]
75. Salavi, P.; Panahandeh, G.; Vatanı, B.; Khoshdel, A. The effect of adding ferrous sulfate to methylphenidate on attention-deficit/hyperactivity disorder in children. *J. Adv. Pharm. Technol. Res.* **2017**, *8*, 138–142. [CrossRef]
76. Rucklidge, J.J.; Eggleston, M.J.; Johnstone, J.M.; Darling, K.; Frampton, C.M. Vitamin-mineral treatment improves aggression and emotional regulation in children with ADHD: A fully blinded, randomized, placebo-controlled trial. *J. Child Psychol. Psychiatry* **2017**, *59*, 232–246. [CrossRef]
77. Cortese, S.; Azoulay, R.; Castellanos, F.; Chalard, F.; Lecendreux, M.; Chechin, D.; Delorme, R.; Sebag, G.; Sbarbati, A.; Mouren, M.-C.; et al. Brain iron levels in attention-deficit/hyperactivity disorder: A pilot MRI study. *World J. Biol. Psychiatry* **2011**, *13*, 223–231. [CrossRef]
78. Lozoff, B. Early Iron Deficiency Has Brain and Behavior Effects Consistent with Dopaminergic Dysfunction. *J. Nutr.* **2011**, *141*, 740S–746S. [CrossRef]
79. Kennedy, D.O. B Vitamins and the Brain: Mechanisms, Dose and Efficacy—A Review. *Nutrients* **2016**, *8*, 68. [CrossRef]
80. Mech, A.W.; Farah, A. Correlation of Clinical Response with Homocysteine Reduction During Therapy with Reduced B Vitamins in Patients with MDD Who Are Positive for MTHFR C677T or A1298C Polymorphism: A randomized, double-blind, place-bo-controlled study. *J. Clin. Psychiatry* **2016**, *77*, 668–671. [CrossRef]
81. Smith, A.D.; Smith, S.; De Jager, C.A.; Whitbread, P.; Johnston, C.; Agacinski, G.; Oulhaj, A.; Bradley, K.M.; Jacoby, R.; Refsum, H. Homocysteine-Lowering by B Vitamins Slows the Rate of Accelerated Brain Atrophy in Mild Cognitive Impairment: A Randomized Controlled Trial. *PLoS ONE* **2010**, *5*, e12244. [CrossRef]

82. Vazir, S.; Nagalla, B.; Thangiah, V.; Kamasamudram, V.; Bhattiprolu, S. Effect of micronutrient supplement on health and nutritional status of schoolchildren: Mental function. *Nutrition* **2006**, *22*, S26–S32. [CrossRef]
83. Arnold, L.E.; Bozzolo, H.; Hollway, J.; Cook, A.; DiSilvestro, R.A.; Bozzolo, D.R.; Crowl, L.; Ramadan, Y.; Williams, C. Serum Zinc Correlates with Parent- and Teacher- Rated Inattention in Children with Attention-Deficit/Hyperactivity Disorder. *J. Child Adolesc. Psychopharmacol.* **2005**, *15*, 628–636. [CrossRef]
84. Cortese, S.; Konofal, E.; Bernardina, B.D.; Mouren, M.-C.; Lecendreux, M. Sleep disturbances and serum ferritin levels in children with attention-deficit/hyperactivity disorder. *Eur. Child Adolesc. Psychiatry* **2009**, *18*, 393–399. [CrossRef]
85. Khan, F.H.; Ahlberg, C.D.; Chow, C.A.; Shah, D.R.; Koo, B.B. Iron, dopamine, genetics, and hormones in the pathophysiology of restless legs syndrome. *J. Neurol.* **2017**, *264*, 1634–1641. [CrossRef]
86. Oner, O.; Oner, P.; Bozkurt, H.; Odabas, E.; Keser, N.; Karadag, H.; Kizilgun, M. Effects of Zinc and Ferritin Levels on Parent and Teacher Reported Symptom Scores in Attention Deficit Hyperactivity Disorder. *Child Psychiatry Hum. Dev.* **2010**, *41*, 441–447. [CrossRef]
87. Swanson, J.M.; Kinsbourne, M.; Nigg, J.; Lanphear, B.; Stefanatos, G.A.; Volkow, N.; Taylor, E.; Casey, B.J.; Castellanos, F.; Wadhwa, P.D. Etiologic Subtypes of Attention-Deficit/Hyperactivity Disorder: Brain Imaging, Molecular Genetic and Environmental Factors and the Dopamine Hypothesis. *Neuropsychol. Rev.* **2007**, *17*, 39–59. [CrossRef]
88. Volkow, N.D.; Wang, G.-J.; Newcorn, J.; Telang, F.; Solanto, M.V.; Fowler, J.S.; Logan, J.; Ma, Y.; Schulz, K.; Pradhan, K.; et al. Depressed Dopamine Activity in Caudate and Preliminary Evidence of Limbic Involvement in Adults With Attention-Deficit/Hyperactivity Disorder. *Arch. Gen. Psychiatry* **2007**, *64*, 932–940. [CrossRef]
89. Bonaventura, J.; Quiroz, C.; Cai, N.-S.; Rubinstein, M.; Tanda, G.; Ferré, S. Key role of the dopamine D 4 receptor in the modulation of corticostriatal glutamatergic neurotransmission. *Sci. Adv.* **2017**, *3*, e1601631. [CrossRef]
90. Unger, E.L.; Bianco, L.E.; Jones, B.C.; Allen, R.P.; Earley, C.J. Low brain iron effects and reversibility on striatal dopamine dynamics. *Exp. Neurol.* **2014**, *261*, 462–468. [CrossRef]
91. Huss, M.; Völp, A.; Stauss-Grabo, M. Supplementation of polyunsaturated fatty acids, magnesium and zinc in children seeking medical advice for attention-deficit/hyperactivity problems—An observational cohort study. *Lipids Health Dis.* **2010**, *9*, 1–12. [CrossRef]
92. Bourre, J.M. Effects of nutrients (in food) on the structure and function of the nervous system: Update on dietary requirements for brain. Part 1: Micronutrients. *J. Nutr. Health Aging* **2006**, *10*, 377–385.
93. Sinn, N.; Wilson, C. Dietary Supplementation with Highly Unsaturated Fatty Acids: Implications for Interventions with Persons with Mental Retardation from Research on Infant Cognitive Development, ADHD, and Other Developmental Disabilities. *Int. Rev. Res. Ment. Retard.* **2006**, 159–196. [CrossRef]
94. Arnold, L.E.; Pinkham, S.M.; Votolato, N. Does Zinc Moderate Essential Fatty Acid and Amphetamine Treatment of Attention-Deficit/Hyperactivity Disorder? *J. Child Adolesc. Psychopharmacol.* **2000**, *10*, 111–117. [CrossRef]
95. Calarge, C.; Farmer, C.; DiSilvestro, R.; Arnold, L.E. Serum Ferritin and Amphetamine Response in Youth with Attention-Deficit/Hyperactivity Disorder. *J. Child Adolesc. Psychopharmacol.* **2010**, *20*, 495–502. [CrossRef]
96. Turner, C.A.; Xie, D.; Zimmerman, B.M. Iron Status in Toddlerhood Predicts Sensitivity to Psychostimulants in Children. *J. Atten. Disord.* **2010**, *16*, 295–303. [CrossRef]
97. Campbell, M.; McKenzie, J.E.; Sowden, A.; Katikireddi, S.V.; Brennan, S.E.; Ellis, S.; Hartmann-Boyce, J.; Ryan, R.; Shepperd, S.; Thomas, J.; et al. Synthesis without meta-analysis (SWiM) in systematic reviews: Reporting guideline. *BMJ* **2020**, *368*, l6890. [CrossRef]

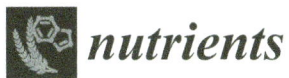

Review

Efficacy and Safety of Polyunsaturated Fatty Acids Supplementation in the Treatment of Attention Deficit Hyperactivity Disorder (ADHD) in Children and Adolescents: A Systematic Review and Meta-Analysis of Clinical Trials

Mina Nicole Händel [1,2,*], Jeanett Friis Rohde [1,2], Marie Louise Rimestad [3], Elisabeth Bandak [1,2], Kirsten Birkefoss [2], Britta Tendal [2], Sanne Lemcke [4] and Henriette Edemann Callesen [2]

[1] The Parker Institute, Bispebjerg and Frederiksberg Hospital, The Capital Region, 2000 Frederiksberg, Denmark; jeanett.friis.rohde@regionh.dk (J.F.R.); elisabeth.ann.bandak@regionh.dk (E.B.)

[2] The Danish Health Authority, 2300 Copenhagen, Denmark; kibi@sst.dk (K.B.); brittatdk@gmail.com (B.T.); henriette.callesen@gmail.com (H.E.C.)

[3] Institute of Psychology, Aarhus University, 8000 Aarhus, Denmark; psykolog-rimestad@protonmail.com

[4] Department of Child and Adolescent Psychiatry, Aarhus University Hospital, Psychiatry, 8200 Aarhus N, Denmark; Sanne.Lemcke@ps.rm.dk

* Correspondence: mina.nicole.holmgaard.handel@regionh.dk

Abstract: Based on epidemiological and animal studies, the rationale for using polyunsaturated fatty acids (PUFAs) as a treatment for Attention Deficit Hyperactivity Disorder (ADHD) seems promising. Here, the objective was to systematically identify and critically assess the evidence from clinical trials. The primary outcome was ADHD core symptoms. The secondary outcomes were behavioral difficulties, quality of life, and side effects. We performed a systematic search in Medline, Embase, Cinahl, PsycInfo, and the Cochrane Library up to June 2020. The overall certainty of evidence was evaluated using Grades of Recommendation, Assessment, Development, and Evaluation (GRADE). We identified 31 relevant randomized controlled trials including 1755 patients. The results showed no effect on ADHD core symptoms rated by parents (k = 23; SMD: −0.17; 95% CI: −0.32, −0.02) or teachers (k = 10; SMD: −0.06; 95% CI: −0.31, 0.19). There was no effect on behavioral difficulties, rated by parents (k = 7; SMD: −0.02; 95% CI: −0.17, 0.14) or teachers (k = 5; SMD: −0.04; 95% CI: −0.35, 0.26). There was no effect on quality of life (SMD: 0.01; 95% CI: −0.29, 0.31). PUFA did not increase the occurrence of side effects. For now, there seems to be no benefit of PUFA in ADHD treatment; however, the certainty of evidence is questionable, and thus no conclusive guidance can be made. The protocol is registered in PROSPERO ID: CRD42020158453.

Keywords: fatty acids; omega 3; polyunsaturated; attention deficit hyperactivity disorder; ADHD; children; adolescents; systematic review; meta-analysis

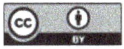

1. Introduction

Attention Deficit Hyperactivity Disorder (ADHD) is a common neurodevelopmental disorder in children and adolescents, which may persist into adulthood. A meta-analysis of 102 prevalence studies found that the worldwide prevalence estimate for ADHD among children and adolescents under the age of 18 years is 3.4% (CI 95% 2.6–4.5) [1].

ADHD is characterized by three core symptoms, namely, inattention, hyperactivity, and impulsivity. The symptoms must be present in different settings and be both impairing and age inappropriate. ADHD is frequently comorbid with other psychiatric disorders and a substantial burden to the affected children and their families [2]. Long-term studies have revealed that a diagnosis of ADHD is associated with lower educational achievements and significant higher prevalence of, e.g., injury, substance abuse, unemployment, and delinquency [3–8].

A wide variety of treatments such as pharmacological and psychosocial interventions are used for the management of ADHD. There is some evidence for the short-term effectiveness of certain non-pharmacological interventions and pharmacological treatments [9–11]. However, some patients and parents are concerned with the use of pharmaceuticals for the treatment of ADHD, and initiation of pharmacological treatment may be linked with a certain degree of reluctance due to side-effects. Investigations of other interventions such as diet or nutritional supplements are therefore necessary.

Based on evidence from epidemiological studies and animal models, the rationale for using polyunsaturated fatty acids (PUFAs) as a treatment option for ADHD is promising. Studies have found that a deficiency of essential fatty acids positively correlates with ADHD symptoms [12]. Supporting the evidence that PUFAs may play a role in brain disorders, essential fatty acids have shown to regulate neurotransmitter and immune functions via the modulation of lipid rafts signaling platforms on the cell membrane in addition to having an anti-inflammatory inhibition of the free radical generation and oxidative stress [13–15].

The objective of this systematic review and meta-analysis was to systematically identify and critically assess the current evidence from clinical trials concerning the administration of supplementation with PUFAs for the treatment of ADHD among children and adolescents (6–18 years). Specifically, we sought to evaluate the effect of supplementation with PUFAs on ADHD core symptoms and behavioral difficulties, rated by both parent and teachers. Furthermore, we sought to investigate the impact on quality of life as well as the occurrence of side effects including diarrhea, gastrointestinal discomfort, and nausea.

The systematic review and meta-analysis were based on an update of the results from a Danish national clinical guideline published in 2018 by the Danish Health Authority.

2. Materials and Methods

Established methods recommended by the Cochrane Collaboration [16] and according to the principles described in the Grades of Recommendation, Assessment, Development, and Evaluation (GRADE) [17] approach were used to conduct this systematic review and meta-analysis. Moreover, the systematic review was structured according to Population, Intervention, Comparison, and Outcome (PICO) characterization [18]. Specifically, the PICO question was whether children and adolescents aged 6–18 years with ADHD should be offered PUFA supplementation. The definitions of population, intervention, comparator, outcomes, and study design are specified in Table 1. The research question is best addressed through a randomized study design in order to evaluate the effectiveness of the intervention so that issues regarding both measured and unmeasured confounding are minimized.

Table 1. Population, Intervention, Comparison, and Outcome (PICO) criteria for inclusion and exclusion of studies.

Population	Children and adolescents between the age of 6 and 18 years (≥ 6 and ≤ 18), diagnosed with ADHD in accordance with ICD-10 or DSM criteria (both 4 and 5) for ADHD.
Intervention	Supplementation of polyunsaturated fatty acids (PUFAs). We included studies investigating both omega 3 and 6 fatty acids.
Comparison	No treatment—placebo and/or regular diet.
Outcome, primary	ADHD core symptoms, parent rated ADHD core symptoms, teacher rated Timing and effect measures ADHD core symptoms, both parent and teacher rated, were investigated at end of treatment. Minimal clinically important difference (MCID) 30% mean total score change difference between treatment groups, which is equivalent to between-treatment difference of 5.2 to 7.7 points [19–21].

Table 1. Cont.

Outcome, secondary	Behavioral difficulties, parent rated Behavioral difficulties, teacher rated Quality of life Diarrhea Gastrointestinal discomfort Nausea Timing and effect measures Behavioral difficulties both parent and teacher rated was investigated at end of treatment. Quality of life was investigated at the longest follow-up time (minimum 3 months after end of treatment). In our published protocol, we initially planned to assess diarrhea, gastrointestinal discomfort, and nausea at longest follow-up. This was later changed to end of treatment, as the identified studies did not provide any follow-up data on these outcomes.
Study design	All randomized controlled studies, with interventions matching the defined research question.

The protocol was registered in the International Prospective Register of Systematic Reviews (PROSPERO: CRD42020158453 (accepted 28 April 2020) and the systematic review was constructed in accordance to the Preferred Reporting Items for Systematic review and Meta-Analysis (PRISMA) statement [22,23] (PRISMA checklist is provided in the Supplementary Material).

2.1. Search Strategy

As a part of the conduct of the Danish national clinical guideline on ADHD by the Danish Health Authority, a literature search were performed by KB in September 2013 (with no restriction on date), in November 2017 (dates restricted to 2013–2017), and again in June 2020 (dates restricted to 2017–2020). The systematic literature search was performed in multiple databases including Medline, Embase, Cinahl, and PsycInfo and limited to randomized controlled trials. The original search strategy included a search for both systematic reviews and individual randomized controlled trials. The justification for the stepwise search strategy is that the Danish Health Authority prioritize to enrich existing guidelines with all available eligible literature approximately every third year. All search strategies for the 2013, 2017, and 2020 searches included medical subject heading (MeSH) and text words related to our eligibility criteria. As an example MeSH terms for the intervention were "unsaturated fatty acid" or "Diet therapy" or "diet supplementation" or "Fish oil" or "Carnitine", or text words for the intervention ((fatty adj1 acid*) or ((Polyunsaturated or poly-unsaturated or unsaturated) adj1 (fat or fatty)) or omega-3 or omega3 or omega 3 or omega-6 or omega6 or omega 6 or (docosahexaenoic adj acid*) or (eicosapentaenoic adj acid*) or (arachidonic adj acid)) or ((fish adj1 oil*) or cod liver oil* or lax oil* or tuna oil* or carnitine or Levocarnitine or "L Carnitine" or L-carnitine or bicarnitine) or ((diet* or food or nutrition) adj1 (therapy or supplement*)) (for further details please see the example presented in Table 2 and in the search protocols provided in Supplementary Material). Both the original and updated searches were limited to literature written in English, Danish, Norwegian, and Swedish due to limitations in language proficiency in the author group. Moreover, to ensure that any relevant studies were not missed by the search, content experts from the guideline working group were conferred with, and reference lists of included articles and previous reviews were screened for potentially relevant studies. Conference abstracts were considered if data were not published elsewhere. Study authors were not contacted to identify additional studies.

Table 2. Example of the search strategy in Embase.

#	Searches
1	exp unsaturated fatty acid/
2	Diet therapy/ or diet supplementation/
3	exp Fish oil/
4	exp Carnitine/
5	((fatty adj1 acid*) or ((Polyunsaturated or poly-unsaturated or unsaturated) adj1 (fat or fatty)) or omega-3 or omega3 or omega 3 or omega-6 or omega6 or omega 6 or (docosahexaenoic adj acid*) or (eicosapentaenoic adj acid*) or (arachidonic adj acid)).ti,ab,kw.
6	((fish adj1 oil*) or cod liver oil* or lax oil* or tuna oil* or carnitine or Levocarnitine or "L Carnitine" or L-carnitine or bicarnitine).ti,ab,kw.
7	((diet* or food or nutrition) adj1 (therapy or supplement*)).ti,ab,kw.
8	or/1–7
9	exp Attention Deficit Disorder/
10	(ADHD or (hyperkinetic adj1 disorder*) or (Attention adj1 Deficit adj1 Disorder) or (attention-deficit adj1 disorder)).ti,ab,kw.
11	9 or 10
12	8 and 11
13	limit 12 to (randomized controlled trial or controlled clinical trial)
14	(((random* or cluster-random* or quasi-random* or control?ed or crossover or cross-over or blind* or mask*) adj4 (trial*1 or study or studies or analy*)) or rct).ti,ab,kw.
15	(placebo* or single-blind* or double-blind* or triple-blind*).ti,ab,kw.
16	((single or double or triple) adj2 (blind* or mask*)).ti,ab,kw.
17	((patient* or person* or participant* or population* or allocat* or assign*) adj3 random*).ti,ab,kw.
18	14 or 15 or 16 or 17
19	12 and 18
20	13 or 19
21	limit 20 to (yr = "2017–2020" and (english or danish or german or norwegian or swedish))

2.2. Study Selection

The search results were imported to RefWorks (Refworks (online software) https://www.refworks.com, accessed on 2 March 2021), and duplicate references were removed. Subsequently, the records were imported into Covidence software (Covidence (Online software)). Covidence team https://www.covidence.org/home, accessed on 2 March 2021) was used for the screening process and data management.

The titles and abstracts of the identified references were screened by one reviewer (MLR), to assess according to the inclusion criteria (Table 1). Subsequently, the full text of potential studies was independently screened by two review authors out of a group of review authors (MLR, SL, HC, JFR, MNH) for eligibility. Disagreement was discussed or by consultation of a third reviewer (BT). Neither of the review authors were blinded to the journal titles, study authors/institutions, or year of publication.

2.3. Extraction of Individual Randomized Controlled Studies

Data extraction was conducted using a predefined template in Covidence software. The assessment of the studies included study settings, population demographics and baseline characteristics, details on intervention and control conditions, study design, outcome, and time of measurement. Two review authors out of a group of review authors (MLR, SL, HC, EB, JFR, MNH) independently extracted data in duplicate. Discrepancies were resolved through discussion in the review team.

Data for analysis were also extracted in Covidence (Online software: https://www.covidence.org/home, accessed on 2 March 2021) and afterwards exported to Review Manager (version 5.2) (Review Manager (RevMan) (Computer program)) (2014). None of the study authors were contacted by email to provide additional information to resolve uncertainties or to obtain missing data. If multiple reports of a single study were identified, the publication with most complete data was included.

2.4. Quality Assessment

Quality assessment of the evidence was evaluated using GRADE method [24]. There are four possible ratings of the quality: high, moderate, low, and very low. Downgrading was carried out for each outcome using the standard definition of risk of bias, inconsistency, indirectness, imprecision, and publication. The overall quality of evidence was based on the lowest quality of the primary outcome and reflected the extent to which we are confident that the effect estimates are correct.

Two review authors out of a group of review authors (MLR, SL, HC, EB, JFR, MNH) independently assessed risk of bias of the primary studies by using the Cochrane risk of bias tool [20] that includes the following characteristics: randomization sequence generation, reatment allocation concealment, blinding of patients and personnel, blinding of outcome assessors, completeness of outcome data, selective outcome reporting, other sources of bias. Discrepancies were resolved through discussion.

2.5. Meta-Analysis

For a dichotomous outcome, the relative risk (RR) was calculated, including the 95% confidence interval (CI). When few or zero events occurred in both the intervention and control group, a risk difference (RD) analysis was performed as sensitivity analysis. For a continuous outcome, since different measurement scales were used, we calculated effect size using the standardized mean difference (SMD), including the 95% confidence interval. Random effect models were used to calculate pooled estimates of effects. Furthermore, a funnel plot was produced to assess the publication bias across the studies, when more than 10 studies were included. Statistical heterogeneity was quantified using I^2 statistic [25], with an I^2 value greater than of 50% considered to be substantial heterogeneity.

Review Manager Software (version 5.3) (The Nordic Cochrane Centre, The Cochrane Collaboration, Copenhagen, Denmark) was used to produce the analyses and forest plots.

3. Results
3.1. Literature Search

In the 2013 search, one systematic review article was found [9], from which 12 randomized trials were identified among the included studies [26–37]. These were supplemented by 11 randomized trials from an updated literature search in 2017 [38–48] and a further eight randomized studies from the latest updated search in 2020 [49–56].

Thus, the evidence base consists of a total of 31 randomized trials.

A flowchart of included secondary and primary studies is presented in Figure 1; Figure 2, and a list of excluded studies after full-text screening including reasons for their exclusion is presented in Supplementary Material.

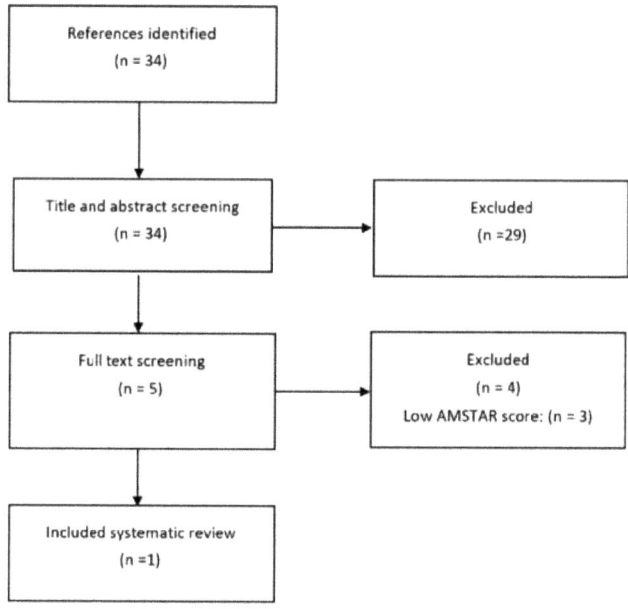

Figure 1. Flowchart of the search for systematic reviews in 2013.

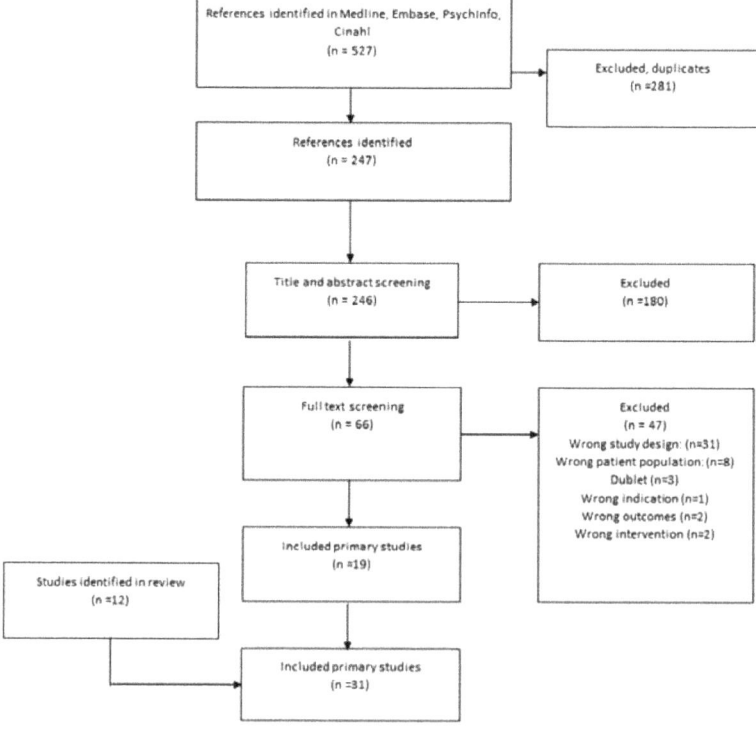

Figure 2. Flowchart of the search for primary studies in 2017 and 2020.

3.2. Review of the Evidence

The populations in the included studies consisted of children with ADHD in the age group ranging from 6–18 years. The interventions consisted of supplements with polyunsaturated fatty acids with either omega 3, omega 6, or combined supplements with both types of fatty acids. The interventions lasted between 8 weeks to 12 months. In some studies [38,49,55], the children were also in medical treatment in both the intervention group and the placebo group, whereby fatty acid treatment was investigated as an active add-on treatment in the intervention group. Information on study identification, baseline characteristics, intervention, control, reported outcomes, and the authors' conclusion is presented in Supplementary Material.

3.2.1. Primary Outcomes

The primary outcomes were reported in 24 studies [29,32,34,35,37–42,44–56] and were based on information from 1755 participants. The results showed no clinically relevant effect was found on the primary outcome parent-rated ADHD core symptoms (SMD: −0.17; 95% CI: −0.32, −0.02) (Figure 3), corresponding to a mean difference on the Parent ADHD rating scale of −1.85 (95% CI: −3.49, −0.22) calculated from the endpoint SD in the control group of Cornu et al., 2018 [51]. The Parent ADHD rating scale ranges from 0 to 54, and thus the result is equivalent to a decrease of 3.4% on the scale (MCID is estimated to a decrease of 30% [19–21]), nor was there any effect found on teacher-rated ADHD core symptoms (k = 10; SMD: −0.06; 95% CI: −0.31, 0.19) [27,29,32,33,35,41,45,50,53] (Figure 4).

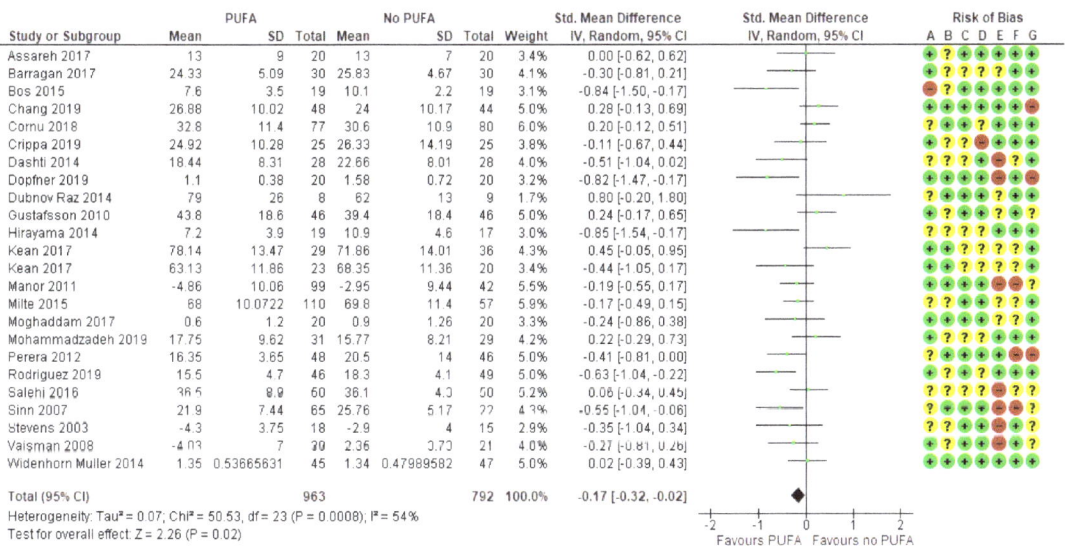

Figure 3. Forest plot of comparison: PUFA vs. placebo, outcome: parent-reported core symptoms (end of treatment). Green square indicates summary estimates of the individual studies. Black diamond indicates total summary effect estimate.

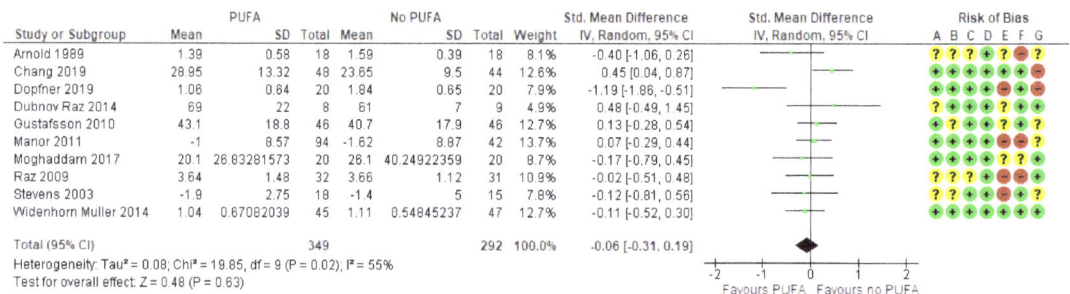

Figure 4. Forest plot of comparison: polyunsaturated fatty acids (PUFA) vs. placebo, outcome: teacher-reported core symptoms (end of treatment). Green square indicates summary estimates of the individual studies. Black diamond indicates total summary effect estimate.

3.2.2. Secondary Outcomes

There was no clinically significant effect on behavioral difficulties, neither when the outcomes were rated by parents (k = 7; SMD: −0.02; 95% CI: −0.17, 0.14) [29,32,35,44,50,52,54] (Figure 5) nor by teachers (k = 5; SMD: −0.04; 95% CI: −0.35, 0.26) [29,32,35,39,50] (Figure 6).

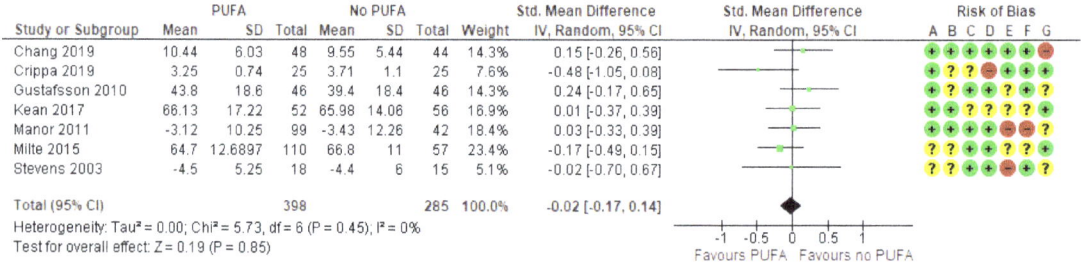

Figure 5. Forest plot of comparison: PUFA vs. placebo, outcome: parent-reported behavioral difficulties (end of treatment). Green square indicates summary estimates of the individual studies. Black diamond indicates total summary effect estimate.

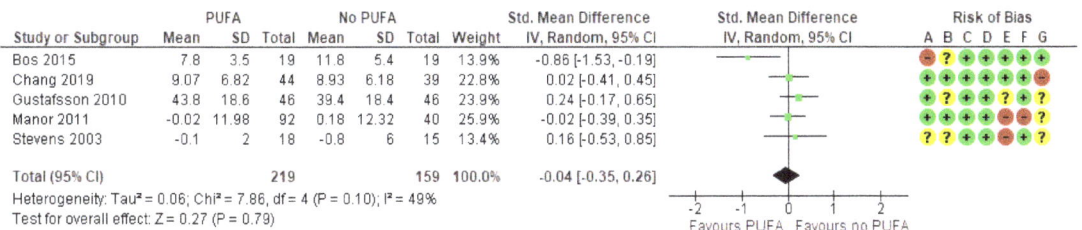

Figure 6. Forest plot of comparison: PUFA vs. placebo, outcome: teacher-reported behavioral difficulties (end of treatment). Green square indicates summary estimates of the individual studies. Black diamond indicates total summary effect estimate.

Only two studies [32,52] examined the effect of the intervention on quality of life, with no significant effect (SMD: 0.01; 95% CI: −0.29, 0.31) (Figure 7).

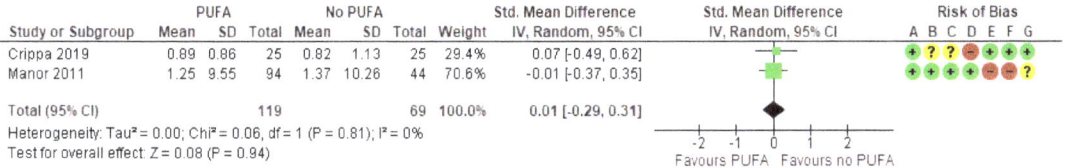

Figure 7. Forest plot of comparison: PUFA vs. placebo, outcome: quality of life (longest follow-up time (minimum 3 months after end of treatment)). Green square indicates summary estimates of the individual studies. Black diamond indicates total summary effect estimate.

Additionally, there were no differences between the intervention group compared to the placebo group regarding the three selected side effects: diarrhea (k = 5, RR: 1.08; 95% CI: 0.32, 3.63 and RD: −0.00; 95% CI: −0.04, 0.03) [29,42,49,50,55], gastrointestinal discomfort (k = 4; RR: 0.72; 95% CI: 0.27, 1.88 and RD: −0.01; 95% CI: −0.04, 0.03) [42–44,55], and nausea (k = 6, RR: 0.99; 95% CI: 0.41, 2.38 and RD: 0.01; 95% CI: −0.02, 0.03) [29,32,33,42,43,49,55] (Figure 8).

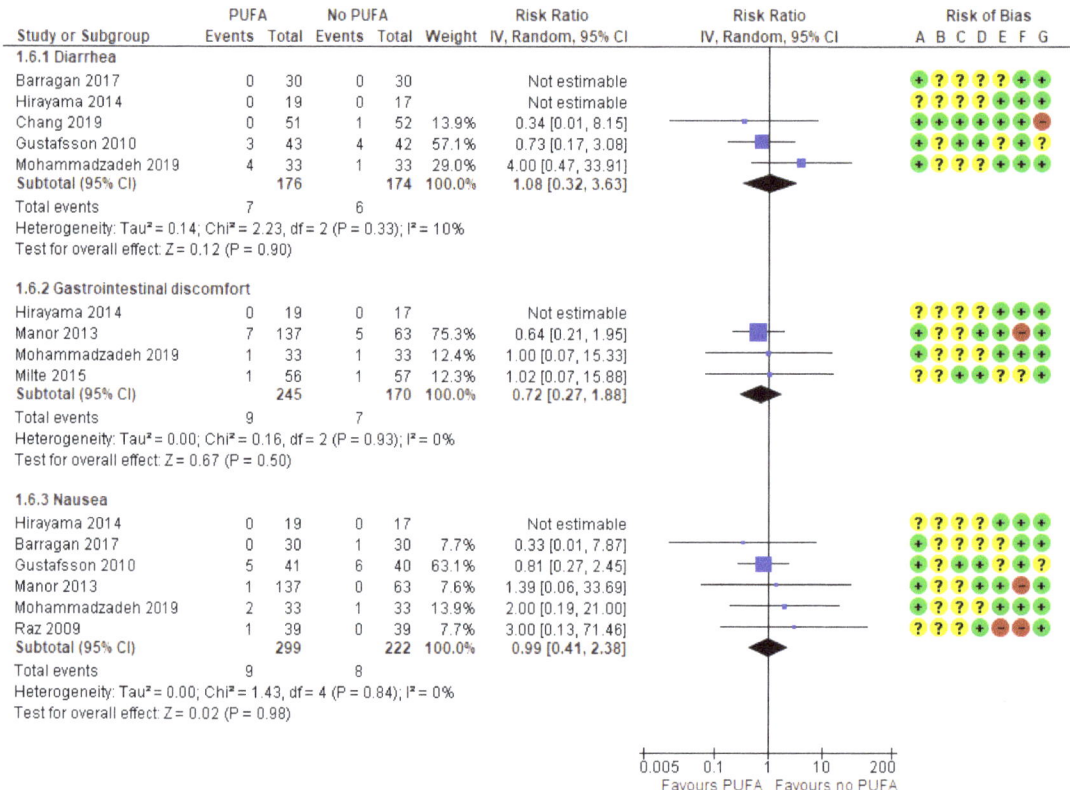

Figure 8. Forest plot of comparison: PUFA vs. placebo, outcome: side effects (end of treatment). Blue square indicates summary estimates of the individual studies. Black diamond indicates total summary effect estimate.

3.3. Certainty of Evidence (GRADE)

The certainty of the evidence was overall low to very low, as there were problems with inaccurate effect estimates in small studies (very serious risk of imprecision) as well as serious risk of bias. The risk of bias was primarily due to problems with blinding of the observers that assessed the effect (parent and teachers). However, the studies generally suffered from methodological flaws and were largely poorly described, especially regarding how the randomization sequence was generated, how the allocation was concealed, and how incomplete data were handled.

4. Discussion

The objective of this systematic literature review and meta-analysis was to provide clinicians, caregivers and guideline panels with an updated overview and critical assessment of the evidence, investigating the effect of PUFA among children aged 6 to 18 years diagnosed with ADHD. Based on a substantial body of evidence, there is no indication that supplementation with PUFA has a positive effect on core symptoms of ADHD, behavioral difficulties, or quality of life. The present review suggests that there is no substantial increase in side effects following the use of PUFA, including the occurrence of diarrhea, gastrointestinal discomfort, or nausea.

Based on our findings, there is insufficient evidence to support patients, parents, clinicians, and caregivers in their decision on whether to use PUFA as a supplementation in the treatment of ADHD. Consequently, the patient preferences are expected to be unambiguous, in the sense that some parents will prefer dietary changes rather than pharmacological treatment, and other parents will find it difficult and relatively intrusive to implement dietary changes in children and adolescents. Effective treatment with PUFA would supposedly depend on the presence of an initial PUFA deficiency observed in the patient at baseline. A significant decrease in PUFA levels has indeed been observed in patients with ADHD as compared to healthy controls [57]. However, it still needs to be investigated what role PUFA plays in the pathology of ADHD. It remains unknown whether PUFA deficiency represents a neuropathological finding directly potentiating symptom outbreak, or rather a compensatory mechanism due to long-standing disease manifestation. In addition, an evaluation of the long-term effects of providing PUFA as a supplement is needed. For now, the effect has only been tested in patients over a time period ranging from 8 weeks to 12 months.

The amount of RCTs investigating the use of PUFA as a treatment for ADHD has increased since the latest Cochrane review by Gilles et al. was published in 2012 [58]. Despite an increase in the number of available studies, the conclusion and quality of the evidence remains unchanged. Thus, the evidence still indicates an inability of PUFA to effectively alter the symptomatology of ADHD. The evidence remains of a low to very low quality, thus reflecting a high degree of uncertainty of the effect estimates.

The risk of bias in the identified studies includes an inadequate random sequence generation and allocation concealment, which in RCTs is mandatory to ensure that intervention and control groups are kept as identical as possible. Thus, the inability to perform sufficient random allocation may induce systematic errors, which may have a considerable impact on the final results. Other major sources of bias were due to incomplete outcome reporting, thus reflecting an increased risk of reporting bias and attrition. Regarding incomplete data, a review has previously described in which problems with drop-out seem to be common in n-3 long chain PUFA supplementation trials in children and adolescents in general [59]. This indicates that dropouts may be a common, inherent issue when seeking to investigate the effect of PUFA in a research setting.

Blinding of the observers evaluating the effect is essential. The included studies generally displayed an unclear level of blinding, as blinding in the majority of studies was inadequately described. Blinding of participants may once again constitute an inherent problem when investigating the effect of PUFA due to the distinct smell and taste [60]. This may unmask the allocation to the respective groups, as patients and parents over time may become aware if they indeed are receiving the active PUFA component. Nevertheless, adequate blinding of observers not directly related to the child should be possible, including the researcher and teachers. Collectively, these problems lead to a high risk of bias, which may essentially have an impact on the results and thereby lead to a distortion in the final conclusion.

Our findings displaying an inadequate effect of PUFA in the treatment of ADHD is in line with many previous reviews on the subject [57,61–65], but not all [66–69].

When comparing our review to others reporting a beneficial effect, it becomes evident that there is a discrepancy in the methodology used to evaluate treatment effects, which may explain the discrepancy in results. In three of the reviews [66,67,69], no specific analysis to obtain pooled estimate of effects was performed, as results from the individual trials were only narratively described. This prevents a direct comparison between trials, including an assessment of the overall magnitude of effect. Common for all reviews reporting a positive effect was a lack of quality assessment of the included studies. This hinders an evaluation of the extent of trust in the data and may essentially mask some issues that otherwise would lead to a downscaling of the certainty in the evidence, and thereby the confidence in the results. It should be mentioned, apart from ADHD core symptoms, the reviews reporting a positive effect also include other outcomes not evaluated in the present review. The inclusion and exclusion criteria furthermore varied across the reviews. This may in part also explain some of the discrepancy in the reported results.

As mentioned above, several inherent methodological issues due indeed exist when it comes to investigating the effect of PUFA in research settings. Nevertheless, this does not unconditionally prevent the possibility of performing high-quality research on the matter. As such, future research should focus on conducting clinical trials of high-quality, following the CONSORT (Consolidated Standards of Reporting Trials) Statement [70]. This is essential if we wish to move forward and be able to conclusively evaluate the role of PUFA in the treatment of ADHD.

Strengths and Limitations of the Current Review

In order to ensure high methodological quality, this systematic review and meta-analyses followed the guidelines of the Cochrane Collaboration and PRISMA as well as pre-registering a protocol at PROSPERO. Moreover, a comprehensive search and duplicate full-text study selection, data extraction, and quality assessment were used. Amongst the limitations, we acknowledge that since the search was limited/restricted to English and Scandinavian languages, there might be relevant studies unidentified. Moreover, grey literature was not searched, and thus relevant studies may have been unidentified. Furthermore, the authors of the included studies were not contacted for further information, and the results are merely based on data published in peer-reviewed articles. The review authors were not blinded in the process of selecting literature.

5. Conclusions

Based on the current low to very low evidence, there seems to be no benefit of providing PUFA supplements to children and adolescents with ADHD concerning parent- or teacher-rated core symptoms, behavioral difficulties, or quality of life. Concerns on adverse effects of PUFA supplementation is limited. Conclusive guidance for patients, parent and clinical practice cannot be made due to the many limitations inherent to the included studies.

Supplementary Materials: The following are available online at https://www.mdpi.com/article/10.3390/nu13041226/s1, Table S1: the Preferred Reporting Items for Systematic review and Meta-Analysis (PRISMA) checklist, Table S2: Search protocol, Table S3: list of excluded studies, Table S4: Study identification of the included randomized controlled trials, Table S5: The baseline characteristic of the included RCTs, Table S6: The intervention, control, reported outcomes, and authors' conclusion of the included RCTs.

Author Contributions: Conceptualization, M.N.H., J.F.R., M.L.R., E.B., K.B., B.T., S.L., H.E.C.; methodology, M.N.H., J.F.R., M.L.R., E.B., K.B., B.T., S.L., H.E.C.; software, not applicable; validation, not applicable; formal analysis, H.E.C.; investigation, M.N.H., J.F.R., M.L.R., E.B., K.B., B.T., S.L., H.E.C.; resources, M.N.H., J.F.R., M.L.R., E.B., K.B., B.T., S.L., H.E.C.; data curation, not applicable; writing—original draft preparation, M.N.H., H.E.C. with contribution from J.F.R., M.L.R., E.B., K.B., B.T., S.L.; writing—review and editing, M.N.H., J.F.R., M.L.R., E.B., K.B., B.T., S.L., H.E.C.; visualization, M.N.H., H.E.C.; supervision, not applicable; project administration, M.N.H., H.E.C.; funding acquisition, M.N.H., J.F.R., M.L.R., E.B., K.B., B.T., S.L., H.E.C. All authors have read and agreed to the published version of the manuscript.

Funding: The study was initiated and financed by the Danish Health Authority. The Parker Institute at Bispebjerg and Frederiksberg Hospital was supported by a core grant from the Oak Foundation (OCAY-13-309).

Institutional Review Board Statement: Not applicable.

Informed Consent Statement: Not applicable.

Data Availability Statement: Data are available at the Danish Health Authority website (www.sst.dk), accessed on 4 April 2021.

Acknowledgments: The study was initiated and financed by the Danish Health Authority. The Parker Institute at Bispebjerg and Frederiksberg Hospital was supported by a core grant from the Oak Foundation (OCAY-13-309). The authors would like to thank the work and reference group, as well as the secretary of the "National Clinical Guideline for the Treatment of ADHD in Children and Adolescents", The Danish Health Authority.

Conflicts of Interest: The authors declare no conflict of interest. The funders had no role in the design of the study; in the collection, analyses, or interpretation of data; in the writing of the manuscript, or in the decision to publish the results.

References

1. Polanczyk, G.V.; Salum, G.A.; Sugaya, L.S.; Caye, A.; Rohde, L.A. Annual research review: A meta-analysis of the worldwide prevalence of mental disorders in children and adolescents. *J. Child Psychol. Psychiatry* **2015**, *56*, 345–365. [CrossRef]
2. Thapar, A.; Cooper, M. Attention deficit hyperactivity disorder. *Lancet* **2016**, *387*, 1240–1250. [CrossRef]
3. Barkley, R.A.; Fischer, M. Hyperactive Child Syndrome and Estimated Life Expectancy at Young Adult Follow-Up: The Role of ADHD Persistence and Other Potential Predictors. *J. Atten. Disord.* **2019**, *23*, 907–923. [CrossRef] [PubMed]
4. Mohr-Jensen, C.; Steinhausen, H.C. A meta-analysis and systematic review of the risks associated with childhood attention-deficit hyperactivity disorder on long-term outcome of arrests, convictions, and incarcerations. *Clin. Psychol. Rev.* **2016**, *48*, 32–42. [CrossRef]
5. Dalsgaard, S.; Leckman, J.F.; Mortensen, P.B.; Nielsen, H.S.; Simonsen, M. Effect of drugs on the risk of injuries in children with attention deficit hyperactivity disorder: A prospective cohort study. *Lancet Psychiatry* **2015**, *2*, 702–709. [CrossRef]
6. Franke, B.; Michelini, G.; Asherson, P.; Banaschewski, T.; Bilbow, A.; Buitelaar, J.K.; Cormand, B.; Faraone, S.V.; Ginsberg, Y.; Haavik, J.; et al. Live fast, die young? A review on the developmental trajectories of ADHD across the lifespan. *Eur. Neuropsychopharmacol.* **2018**, *28*, 1059–1088. [CrossRef]
7. Galera, C.; Melchior, M.; Chastang, J.F.; Bouvard, M.P.; Fombonne, E. Childhood and adolescent hyperactivity-inattention symptoms and academic achievement 8 years later: The GAZEL Youth study. *Psychol. Med.* **2009**, *39*, 1895–1906. [CrossRef]
8. Erskine, H.E.; Norman, R.E.; Ferrari, A.J.; Chan, G.C.; Copeland, W.E.; Whiteford, H.A.; Scott, J.G. Long-Term Outcomes of Attention-Deficit/Hyperactivity Disorder and Conduct Disorder: A Systematic Review and Meta-Analysis. *J. Am. Acad. Child Adolesc. Psychiatry* **2016**, *55*, 841–850. [CrossRef]
9. Sonuga-Barke, E.J.; Brandeis, D.; Cortese, S.; Daley, D.; Ferrin, M.; Holtmann, M.; Stevenson, J.; Danckaerts, M.; Van der Oord, S.; Döpfner, M.; et al. Nonpharmacological interventions for ADHD: Systematic review and meta-analyses of randomized controlled trials of dietary and psychological treatments. *Am. J. Psychiatry* **2013**, *170*, 275–289. [CrossRef]
10. De, C.F.; Cortese, S.; Adamo, N.; Janiri, L. Pharmacological and non-pharmacological treatment of adults with ADHD: A meta-review. *Evid. Based Ment. Health* **2017**, *20*, 4–11.
11. Storebø, O.J.; Krogh, H.B.; Ramstad, E.; Moreira-Maia, C.R.; Holmskov, M.; Skoog, M.; Nilausen, T.D.; Magnusson, F.L.; Zwi, M.; Gillies, D.; et al. Methylphenidate for attention-deficit/hyperactivity disorder in children and adolescents: Cochrane systematic review with meta-analyses and trial sequential analyses of randomised clinical trials. *BMJ* **2015**, *351*, h5203. [CrossRef] [PubMed]
12. Chang, J.P.-C.; Jingling, L.; Huang, Y.-T.; Lu, Y.-J.; Su, K.-P. Delay Aversion, Temporal Processing, and N-3 Fatty Acids Intake in Children with Attention-Deficit/Hyperactivity Disorder (ADHD). *Clin. Psychol. Sci.* **2016**, *4*, 1094–1103. [CrossRef]
13. Haag, M. Essential fatty acids and the brain. *Can. J. Psychiatry* **2003**, *48*, 195–203. [CrossRef]
14. Yaqoob, P.; Calder, P.C. Fatty acids and immune function: New insights into mechanisms. *Br. J. Nutr.* **2007**, *98* (Suppl. 1), S41–S45. [CrossRef]
15. Simopoulos, A.P. Essential fatty acids in health and chronic diseases. *Forum Nutr.* **2003**, *56*, 67–70. [CrossRef]
16. Higgins, J.P.T.; Green, S. Assessing risk of bias in cross-over trials. In *Cochrane Handbook of Systematic Reviews of Interventions*; The Cochrane Collaboration Version 5.1.0; John Wiley & Sons: Chichester, UK, 2011.
17. Guyatt, G.H.; Oxman, A.D.; Schunemann, H.J.; Tugwell, P.; Knottnerus, A. GRADE guidelines: A new series of articles in the Journal of Clinical Epidemiology. *J. Clin. Epidemiol.* **2011**, *64*, 380–382. [CrossRef] [PubMed]
18. Guyatt, G.H.; Oxman, A.D.; Kunz, R.; Atkins, D.; Brozek, J.; Vist, G.; Alderson, P.; Glasziou, P.; Falck-Ytter, Y.; Schünemann, H.J. GRADE guidelines: 2. Framing the question and deciding on important outcomes. *J. Clin. Epidemiol.* **2011**, *64*, 395–400. [CrossRef] [PubMed]
19. Canadian Agency for Drugs and Technologies in Health. *Guanfacine Hydrochloride Extended Release (Intuniv XR) Tablets: For the Treatment of Attention-Deficit/Hyperactivity Disorder [Internet]: Appendix 5: Validity of Outcome Measures*; Canadian Agency for Drugs and Technologies in Health: Ottawa, ON, Canada, 2015.
20. Zhang, S.; Faries, D.E.; Vowles, M.; Michelson, D. ADHD Rating Scale IV: Psychometric properties from a multinational study as a clinician-administered instrument. *Int. J. Methods Psychiatr. Res.* **2005**, *14*, 186–201. [CrossRef]
21. Buitelaar, J.K.; Montgomery, S.A.; van Zwieten-Boot, B.J. Attention deficit hyperactivity disorder: Guidelines for investigating efficacy of pharmacological intervention. *Eur. Neuropsychopharmacol.* **2003**, *13*, 297–304. [CrossRef]

22. Liberati, A.; Altman, D.G.; Tetzlaff, J.; Mulrow, C.; Gøtzsche, P.C.; Ioannidis, J.P.; Clarke, M.; Devereaux, P.J.; Kleijnen, J.; Moher, D. The PRISMA statement for reporting systematic reviews and meta-analyses of studies that evaluate health care interventions: Explanation and elaboration. *J. Clin. Epidemiol.* **2009**, *62*, e1–e34. [CrossRef]
23. Moher, D.; Shamseer, L.; Clarke, M.; Ghersi, D.; Liberati, A.; Petticrew, M. Preferred reporting items for systematic review and meta-analysis protocols (PRISMA-P) 2015 statement. *Syst. Rev.* **2015**, *4*, 1. [CrossRef]
24. Guyatt, G.; Oxman, A.D.; Akl, E.A.; Kunz, R.; Vist, G.; Brozek, J.; Norris, S.; Falck-Ytter, Y.; Glasziou, P.; DeBeer, H.; et al. GRADE guidelines: 1. Introduction-GRADE evidence profiles and summary of findings tables. *J. Clin. Epidemiol.* **2011**, *64*, 383–394. [CrossRef]
25. Higgins, J.P.; Thompson, S.G. Quantifying heterogeneity in a meta-analysis. *Stat. Med.* **2002**, *21*, 1539–1558. [CrossRef] [PubMed]
26. Aman, M.G.; Mitchell, E.A.; Turbott, S.H. The effects of essential fatty acid supplementation by Efamol in hyperactive children. *J. Abnorm. Child Psychol.* **1987**, *15*, 75–90. [CrossRef]
27. Arnold, L.E.; Kleykamp, D.; Votolato, N.A.; Taylor, W.A.; Kontras, S.B.; Tobin, K. Gamma-linolenic acid for attention-deficit hyperactivity disorder: Placebo-controlled comparison to D-amphetamine. *Biol. Psychiatry* **1989**, *25*, 222–228. [CrossRef]
28. Bélanger, S.A.; Vanasse, M.; Spahis, S.; Sylvestre, M.P.; Lippé, S.; l'Heureux, F.; Ghadirian, P.; Vanasse, C.M.; Levy, E. Omega-3 fatty acid treatment of children with attention-deficit hyperactivity disorder: A randomized, double-blind, placebo-controlled study. *Paediatr. Child Health* **2009**, *14*, 89–98. [CrossRef]
29. Gustafsson, P.A.; Birberg-Thornberg, U.; Duchén, K.; Landgren, M.; Malmberg, K.; Pelling, H.; Strandvik, B.; Karlsson, T. EPA supplementationn improves teacher-rated behaviour and oppositional symptoms in children with ADHD. *Acta Paediatr.* **2010**, *99*, 1540–1549. [CrossRef]
30. Johnson, M.; Ostlund, S.; Fransson, G.; Kadesjo, B.; Gillberg, C. Omega-3/omega-6 fatty acids for attention deficit hyperactivity disorder: A randomized placebo-controlled trial in children and adolescents. *J. Atten. Disord.* **2009**, *12*, 394–401. [CrossRef]
31. Hirayama, S.; Hamazaki, T.; Terasawa, K. Effect of docosahexaenoic acid-containing food administration on symptoms of attention-deficit/hyperactivity disorder—a placebo-controlled double-blind study. *Eur. J. Clin. Nutr.* **2004**, *58*, 467–473. [CrossRef]
32. Manor, I.; Magen, A.; Keidar, D.; Rosen, S.; Tasker, H.; Cohen, T.; Richter, Y.; Zaaroor-Regev, D.; Manor, Y.; Weizman, A. The effect of phosphatidylserine containing Omega3 fatty-acids on attention-deficit hyperactivity disorder symptoms in children: A double-blind placebo-controlled trial, followed by an open-label extension. *Eur. Psychiatry* **2012**, *27*, 335–342. [CrossRef]
33. Raz, R.; Carasso, R.L.; Yehuda, S. The influence of short-chain essential fatty acids on children with attention-deficit/hyperactivity disorder: A double-blind placebo-controlled study. *J. Child Adolesc. Psychopharmacol.* **2009**, *19*, 167–177. [CrossRef]
34. Sinn, N.; Bryan, J. Effect of supplementation with polyunsaturated fatty acids and micronutrients on learning and behavior problems associated with child ADHD. *J. Dev. Behav. Pediatr.* **2007**, *28*, 82–91. [CrossRef]
35. Stevens, L.; Zhang, W.; Peck, L.; Kuczek, T.; Grevstad, N.; Mahon, A.; Zentall, S.S.; Eugene Arnold, L.; Burgess, J.R. EFA supplementation in children with inattention, hyperactivity, and other disruptive behaviors. *Lipids* **2003**, *38*, 1007–1021. [CrossRef]
36. Voigt, R.G.; Llorente, A.M.; Jensen, C.L.; Fraley, J.K.; Berretta, M.C.; Heird, W.C. A randomized, double-blind, placebo-controlled trial of docosahexaenoic acid supplementation in children with attention-deficit/hyperactivity disorder. *J. Pediatr.* **2001**, *139*, 189–196. [CrossRef]
37. Vaisman, N.; Kaysar, N.; Zaruk-Adasha, Y.; Pelled, D.; Brichon, G.; Zwingelstein, G.; Bodennec, J. Correlation between changes in blood fatty acid composition and visual sustained attention performance in children with inattention: Effect of dietary n-3 fatty acids containing phospholipids. *Am. J. Clin. Nutr.* **2008**, *87*, 1170–1180. [CrossRef]
38. Assareh, M.; Davari Ashtiani, R.; Khademi, M.; Jazayeri, S.; Rai, A.; Nikoo, M. Efficacy of Polyunsaturated Fatty Acids (PUFA) in the Treatment of Attention Deficit Hyperactivity Disorder. *J. Atten. Disord.* **2017**, *21*, 78–85. [CrossRef]
39. Bos, D.J.; Oranje, B.; Veerhoek, E.S.; Van Diepen, R.M.; Weusten, J.M.; Demmelmair, H.; Koletzko, B.; Eilander, A.; Hoeksma, M.; Durston, S. Reduced Symptoms of Inattention after Dietary Omega-3 Fatty Acid Supplementation in Boys with and without Attention Deficit/Hyperactivity Disorder. *Neuropsychopharmacology* **2015**, *40*, 2298–2306. [CrossRef]
40. Dashti, N.; Hekmat, H.; Soltani, H.R.; Rahimdel, A.; Javaherchian, M. Comparison of therapeutic effects of omega-3 and methylphenidate (ritalin®) in treating children with attention deficit hyperactivity disorder. *Iran. J. Psychiatry Behav. Sci.* **2014**, *8*, 7.
41. Dubnov-Raz, G.; Khoury, Z.; Wright, I.; Raz, R.; Berger, I. The effect of alpha-linolenic acid supplementation on ADHD symptoms in children: A randomized controlled double-blind study. *Front. Hum. Neurosci.* **2014**, *8*, 780. [CrossRef]
42. Hirayama, S.; Terasawa, K.; Rabeler, R.; Hirayama, T.; Inoue, T.; Tatsumi, Y.; Purpura, M.; Jäger, R. The effect of phosphatidylserine administration on memory and symptoms of attention-deficit hyperactivity disorder: A randomised, double-blind, placebo-controlled clinical trial. *J. Hum. Nutr. Diet.* **2014**, *27*, 284–291. [CrossRef]
43. Manor, I.; Magen, A.; Keidar, D.; Rosen, S.; Tasker, H.; Cohen, T.; Richter, Y.; Zaaroor-Regev, D.; Manor, Y.; Weizman, A. Safety of phosphatidylserine containing omega3 fatty acids in ADHD children: A double-blind placebo-controlled trial followed by an open-label extension. *Eur. Psychiatry* **2013**, *28*, 386–391. [CrossRef]
44. Milte, C.M.; Parletta, N.; Buckley, J.D.; Coates, A.M.; Young, R.M.; Howe, P.R.C. Increased Erythrocyte Eicosapentaenoic Acid and Docosahexaenoic Acid Are Associated with Improved Attention and Behavior in Children With ADHD in a Randomized Controlled Three-Way Crossover Trial. *J. Atten. Disord.* **2015**, *19*, 954–964. [CrossRef]
45. Moghaddam, M.F.; Shamekhi, M.; Rakhshani, T. Effectiveness of methylphenidate and PUFA for the treatment of patients with ADHD: A double-blinded randomized clinical trial. *Electron. Physician* **2017**, *9*, 4412. [CrossRef] [PubMed]

46. Salehi, B.; Mohammadbeigi, A.; Sheykholeslam, H.; Moshiri, E.; Dorreh, F. Omega-3 and Zinc supplementation as complementary therapies in children with attention-deficit/hyperactivity disorder. *J. Res. Pharm. Pract.* **2016**, *5*, 22.
47. Widenhorn-Muller, K.; Schwanda, S.; Scholz, E.; Spitzer, M.; Bode, H. Effect of supplementation with long-chain omega-3 polyunsaturated fatty acids on behavior and cognition in children with attention deficit/hyperactivity disorder (ADHD): A randomized placebo-controlled intervention trial. *Prostaglandins Leukot. Essent. Fat. Acids* **2014**, *91*, 49–60. [CrossRef] [PubMed]
48. Perera, H.; Jeewandara, K.C.; Seneviratne, S.; Guruge, C. Combined omega3 and omega6 supplementation in children with attention-deficit hyperactivity disorder (ADHD) refractory to methylphenidate treatment: A double-blind, placebo-controlled study. *J. Child Neurol.* **2012**, *27*, 747–753. [CrossRef] [PubMed]
49. Barragan, E.; Breuer, D.; Dopfner, M. Efficacy and Safety of Omega-3/6 Fatty Acids, Methylphenidate, and a Combined Treatment in Children with ADHD. *J. Atten. Disord.* **2017**, *21*, 433–441. [CrossRef]
50. Chang, J.P.C.; Su, K.P.; Mondelli, V.; Satyanarayanan, S.K.; Yang, H.T.; Chiang, Y.J.; Chen, H.T.; Pariante, C.M. High-dose eicosapentaenoic acid (EPA) improves attention and vigilance in children and adolescents with attention deficit hyperactivity disorder (ADHD) and low endogenous EPA levels. *Transl. Psychiatry* **2019**, *9*, 1–9. [CrossRef] [PubMed]
51. Cornu, C.; Mercier, C.; Ginhoux, T.; Masson, S.; Mouchet, J.; Nony, P.; Kassai, B.; Laudy, V.; Berquin, P.; Franc, N.; et al. A double-blind placebo-controlled randomised trial of omega-3 supplementation in children with moderate ADHD symptoms. *Eur. Child Adolesc. Psychiatry* **2018**, *27*, 377–384. [CrossRef]
52. Crippa, A.; Tesei, A.; Sangiorgio, F.; Salandi, A.; Trabattoni, S.; Grazioli, S.; Agostoni, C.; Molteni, M.; Nobile, M. Behavioral and cognitive effects of docosahexaenoic acid in drug-naive children with attention-deficit/hyperactivity disorder: A randomized, placebo-controlled clinical trial. *Eur. Child Adolesc. Psychiatry* **2019**, *28*, 571–583. [CrossRef]
53. Dopfner, M.; Dose, C.; Breuer, D.; Heintz, S.; Schiffhauer, S.; Banaschewski, T. Efficacy of Omega-3/Omega-6 Fatty Acids in Preschool Children at Risk of ADHD: A Randomized Placebo-Controlled Trial. *J. Atten. Disord.* **2019**. [CrossRef] [PubMed]
54. Kean, J.D.; Sarris, J.; Scholey, A.; Silberstein, R.; Downey, L.A.; Stough, C. Reduced inattention and hyperactivity and improved cognition after marine oil extract (PCSO-524 R) supplementation in children and adolescents with clinical and subclinical symptoms of attention-deficit hyperactivity disorder (ADHD): A randomised, double-blind, placebo-controlled trial. *Psychopharmacology* **2017**, *234*, 403–420. [PubMed]
55. Mohammadzadeh, S.; Baghi, N.; Yousefi, F.; Yousefzamani, B. Effect of omega-3 plus methylphenidate as an alternative therapy to reduce attention deficit-hyperactivity disorder in children. *Korean J. Pediatr.* **2019**, *62*, 360. [CrossRef]
56. Rodriguez, C.; Garcia, T.; Areces, D.; Fernandez, E.; Garcia-Noriega, M.; Domingo, J.C. Supplementation with high-content docosahexaenoic acid triglyceride in attention-deficit hyperactivity disorder: A randomized double-blind placebo-controlled trial. *Neuropsychiatr. Dis. Treat.* **2019**, *15*, 1193. [CrossRef]
57. Tesei, A.; Crippa, A.; Ceccarelli, S.B.; Mauri, M.; Molteni, M.; Agostoni, C.; Nobile, M. The potential relevance of docosahexaenoic acid and eicosapentaenoic acid to the etiopathogenesis of childhood neuropsychiatric disorders. *Eur. Child Adolesc. Psychiatry* **2017**, *26*, 1011–1030. [CrossRef]
58. Gillies, D.; Sinn, J.K.; Lad, S.S.; Leach, M.J.; Ross, M.J. Polyunsaturated fatty acids (PUFA) for attention deficit hyperactivity disorder (ADHD) in children and adolescents. *Cochrane Database Syst. Rev.* **2012**, *10*, CD007986. [CrossRef]
59. van der Wurff, I.S.M.; Meyer, B.J.; de Groot, R.H.M. Effect of Omega-3 Long Chain Polyunsaturated Fatty Acids (n-3 LCPUFA) Supplementation on Cognition in Children and Adolescents: A Systematic Literature Review with a Focus on n-3 LCPUFA Blood Values and Dose of DHA and EPA. *Nutrients* **2020**, *12*, 3115. [CrossRef]
60. Schachter, H.; Kourad, K.; Meraki, Z.; Lumb, A.; Tran, K.; Miguelez, M. *Effects of Omega-3 FattyAcids on Mental Health. Evidence Report/TechnologyAssessment No 116 (Publication No 05-E022-2)*; Agency for Healthcare Research and Quality: Rockville, MD, USA, 2005.
61. Pelsser, L.M.; Frankena, K.; Toorman, J.; Rodrigues, P.R. Diet and ADHD, Reviewing the Evidence: A Systematic Review of Meta-Analyses of Double-Blind Placebo-Controlled Trials Evaluating the Efficacy of Diet Interventions on the Behavior of Children with ADHD. *PLoS ONE* **2017**, *12*, e0169277. [CrossRef] [PubMed]
62. Lange, K.W.; Hauser, J.; Lange, K.M.; Makulska-Gertruda, E.; Nakamura, Y.; Reissmann, A.; Sakaue, Y.; Takano, T.; Takeuchi, Y. The Role of Nutritional Supplements in the Treatment of ADHD: What the Evidence Says. *Curr. Psychiatry Rep.* **2017**, *19*, 8. [CrossRef]
63. Catalá-López, F.; Hutton, B.; Núñez-Beltrán, A.; Page, M.J.; Ridao, M.; Macías Saint-Gerons, D.; Catalá, M.A.; Tabarés-Seisdedos, R.; Moher, D. The pharmacological and non-pharmacological treatment of attention deficit hyperactivity disorder in children and adolescents: A systematic review with network meta-analyses of randomised trials. *PLoS ONE* **2017**, *12*, e0180355. [CrossRef] [PubMed]
64. Banaschewski, T.; Belsham, B.; Bloch, M.H.; Ferrin, M.; Johnson, M.; Kustow, J.; Robinson, S.; Zuddas, A. Supplementation with polyunsaturated fatty acids (PUFAs) in the management of attention deficit hyperactivity disorder (ADHD). *Nutr. Health* **2018**, *24*, 279–284. [CrossRef] [PubMed]
65. Perez Carmona, M.P. Complementary/alternative medicine in adolescents with attention deficit hyperactivity disorder and mood disorders. *Rev. Chil. Pediatr.* **2017**, *88*, 294–299.
66. Derbyshire, E. Do Omega-3/6 Fatty Acids Have a Therapeutic Role in Children and Young People with ADHD? *J. Lipids* **2017**, *2017*, 6285218. [CrossRef]

67. Chang, J.P.; Su, K.P. Nutritional Neuroscience as Mainstream of Psychiatry: The Evidence- Based Treatment Guidelines for Using Omega-3 Fatty Acids as a New Treatment for Psychiatric Disorders in Children and Adolescents. *Clin. Psychopharmacol. Neurosci.* **2020**, *18*, 469–483. [CrossRef]
68. Chang, J.P.; Su, K.P.; Mondelli, V.; Pariante, C.M. Omega-3 Polyunsaturated Fatty Acids in Youths with Attention Deficit Hyperactivity Disorder: A Systematic Review and Meta-Analysis of Clinical Trials and Biological Studies. *Neuropsychopharmacology* **2018**, *43*, 534–545. [CrossRef] [PubMed]
69. Heilskov Rytter, M.J.; Andersen, L.B.B.; Houmann, T.; Bilenberg, N.; Hvolby, A.; Mølgaard, C.; Michaelsen, K.F.; Lauritzen, L. Diet in the treatment of ADHD in children—a systematic review of the literature. *Nord. J. Psychiatry* **2015**, *69*, 1–18. [CrossRef] [PubMed]
70. Turner, L.; Shamseer, L.; Altman, D.G.; Weeks, L.; Peters, J.; Kober, T.; Dias, S.; Schulz, K.F.; Plint, A.C.; Moher, D. Consolidated standards of reporting trials (CONSORT) and the completeness of reporting of randomised controlled trials (RCTs) published in medical journals. *Cochrane Database Syst. Rev.* **2012**, *11*, MR000030. [CrossRef]

MDPI
St. Alban-Anlage 66
4052 Basel
Switzerland
Tel. +41 61 683 77 34
Fax +41 61 302 89 18
www.mdpi.com

Nutrients Editorial Office
E-mail: nutrients@mdpi.com
www.mdpi.com/journal/nutrients

www.ingramcontent.com/pod-product-compliance
Lightning Source LLC
LaVergne TN
LVHW070613100526
838202LV00012B/640